How to become an E~~arly~~

The easy way to be up with the ~~larks, using~~
morning routines and better sleep habits – with lots
of practical tips

©2020, Lutz Schneider

Expertengruppe Verlag

The contents of this book have been written with great care. However, we cannot guarantee the accuracy, comprehensiveness and topicality of the subject matter. The contents of the book represent the personal experiences and opinions of the author. No legal responsibility or liability will be accepted for damages caused by counter-productive practices or errors of the reader. There is also no guarantee of success. The author, therefore, does not accept responsibility for lack of success, using the methods described in this book.

All information contained herein is purely for information purposes. It does not represent a recommendation or application of the methods mentioned within. This book does not purport to be complete, nor can the topicality and accuracy of the book be guaranteed. This book in no way replaces the competent recommendations of, or care given by a doctor. The author and publisher do not take responsibility for inconvenience or damages caused by use of the information contained herein.

How to become an Early Bird

The easy way to be up with the larks, using new morning routines and better sleep habits – with lots of practical tips

Publisher: Expertengruppe Verlag

CONTENTS

About the author 8
Preface 10
The internal clock 17
   Der circadian rhythm 18
   Sleep-wake rhythm 20
      What happens in the body? 21
      External influences 23
      Dysfunctions 24
   A feeling for time 25
   Living out of step with the biological rhythm 29
Sleep 31
   Why do we sleep? 33
      Processing Information 34
      Regeneration of the cardio-vascular system 35
      Regulating the metabolism 36
      Strengthening the immune system 37
      Release of grown hormones 38
      Resting the mind 39

- The 5 phases of sleep 40
  - 1st sleep phase: Falling asleep (Non-REM Phase) 41
  - 2nd Sleep phase: Light sleep phase (Non-REM Phase) 42
  - 3rd and 4th Sleep phase: The deep sleep phase (Non-REM Phase) 43
  - 5th Sleep phase: The dream sleep – Die REM Phase 45
- Sleeping cycles 47
  - Waking up at night 49
- Length of sleep 51
- Sleep deficit 53
  - Origins of sleep deficit 54
  - Consequences 57
- 8 Tips for better sleep 59
- Owls and larks 63
  - Larks: Early birds 64
  - Owls: Late risers 66
  - Who is more successful? 68

- Self test 72
  - The Test 73
  - Scores 76
- Morning routine 78
  - Reasons why it is worth using those early morning hours. 80
  - The most common mistakes in the morning routine 83
  - What helps you to get up in the morning? 89
- Food and drink 94
  - Caffeine 95
    - Theanine or caffeine in tea? 98
  - Alcohol 99
  - Rules for a good breakfast 101
    - Rule 1: Wholegrain 103
    - Rule 2: Reduce sugar 104
    - Rule 3: Reduce unhealthy fat 105
    - Healthy alternatives 106
  - Nutrition tips for healthy sleep 109

When to eat 110

A nap after lunch? 111

When and what to eat 112

When should I drink my last caffeine-containing beverage? 113

Which teas/herbal infusions induce sleep? 114

Is a bedtime sweet allowed? 115

Activating body and mind 116

Early morning sport 117

A 10 Minute morning exercise 118

Relaxation techniques 125

The sun salutation 126

Five motivation tips 134

Use the quiet time 135

Boost your metabolism 136

Discipline 137

Be successful 138

Feeling happy all day 139

The early bird challenge in 10 steps 140

Step 1: Find a reason to get up in the morning .. 142

Step 2: Find your new sleeping rhythm 145

    Sleep less through correct sleep 146

Step 3: Establish your morning routine 149

    S.A.V.E.R. by Elrod 150

Step 4: Define your evening routine 153

    Tips to calm down in the evening 154

Step 5: Preparation is everything 158

Step 6: Optimise your alarm system 159

Step 7: Get straight out of bed 160

Step 8: Plan your weekends meaningfully 161

Step 9: Keep at it! 162

Step 10: Enjoy your new life as an early bird 165

Conclusion 166

Did you enjoy my book? 170

Book Recommendations 172

List of references 178

Disclaimer 183

ABOUT THE AUTHOR

Lutz Schneider lives with his wife, Doris, in an old farmhouse in beautiful Rhineland.

Ever since he studied the biology of evolution, over 20 years ago, he has been interested in marginal health subjects, which are often hidden from the main stream, but which are scientifically well accepted. He teaches this knowledge, not only to his students, but also reaches a wider audience in Germany with his various publications.

In his books, he speaks about subjects, the positive effects of which are widely unknown and on which he can pass on his own experiences. All of his publications, therefore, are based on indisputable scientific facts, but also encompass his own very personal experiences and knowledge. This way, the reader not only receives factual information about the subject but also a practical guide with a wide range of knowledge and useful tips, which are easy to understand and put into practice.

Lutz Schneider's easy to read work puts the reader into a relaxed and pleasant ambience, while gaining insight into a subject which few know anything about but which everyone could profit from.

PREFACE

Starting of the day effortlessly, doing things which are good for you; things which you hardly have time for in everyday life, so that you can go to work each day with a deep inner calm: Does that sound like a perfect start to the day? Exactly! Mornings have so much more to offer than tiredness and bad moods. But is it possible for every type of sleeper – whether early morning or late-night people – to use the early hours of the day in a positive way?

Do you belong to the type of person who would rather turn off the alarm in the mornings and not get up at all? I can understand that well, I used to be like that until I became an early bird. But just like you, I made the decision that I wanted to change that. I wanted to be more successful, to achieve more and look back more positively on the day which had just passed.

I often work in my home office. On such days, I found it really difficult to get out of bed. The thought, that I needed to start work immediately, did not exactly do anything for my motivation. So I got up and slowly got myself into gear. I felt anything but fresh and my concentration was not very good either.

Naturally, I did not manage to get all my work done and ended up having to catch up in the evenings. My good intention to do more sport also ended up as no more than a dream. I became frustrated. I started looking for a strategy, which would enable me to get more out of my days. It may seem obvious that you need to get up early, if you want to get more out of your day. There is probably something in the saying: "The early bird catches the worm". Many well-known people are early birds. But how do you become one?

I started to go earlier to bed each evening. It was my aim to be in bed by 10.30pm each evening and to rise at 7am. In comparison: I did not use to go to bed until after midnight and sometimes slept until 9am. The first few days, I was lying wide awake in bed, tossing and turning. I was not going to sleep any earlier and, in the morning, I was not rested. Despite that, I forced myself out of bed, feeling tired and not really ready for anything, as I had hoped for. After a few days, I was managing to go to bed between 10.15pm and 10.30pm, because getting up early in the morning was indeed making me tired. Nevertheless, I did not feel fitter during the day and getting up remained an ordeal. After a few days, I gave up and went back to my old habits, including my discontent.

However, I could not get rid of the idea of getting up early instead of sleeping in. I started to look into the subject of sleep, different types of sleepers and morning routines. During my research, I came across some interesting facts, which I did not know about during my first attempt. With my new knowledge, I made a second attempt, using a new method. The most interesting thing about it all for me was, that I could get up better with less sleep than on my first attempt. Instead of going to bed at 10.30pm I did not go until 11.15pm. I still set my alarm for 7am. Why did that work better? I set my sleeping time according to my sleep phases. During the first trial, I was probably waking myself up during my deepest sleep and that made getting up an ordeal. On the second trial, I adapted my sleep behaviour to my biological rhythm and, how about that, it worked! I was able to wake up much more easily and I was ready for anything.

The problem of not being tired at night was, of course, not solved. However, with a few slight changes to my routine, I was able to get to sleep much more quickly. One important factor in changing my routine was to avoid using electronics with screens, such as my TV, laptop and smartphone. Without exaggeration, I was happy to sit in front of my TV with my laptop on my knee and my smartphone in my hand. There was too much information going into my brain at night, and too much blue light, which was disturbing my hormone production.

I started to concentrate more on my books. I do actually like to read but have not had much time for it lately because – as I said – I was busy doing other things which, in hindsight, were not good for me.

These changes to my evening routine really helped me to successfully complete my 30-day early bird challenge. In addition to changing my evening routine, this time I also made some changes to my morning routine. Whilst lying in bed in the evening I knew exactly what I would do, in which order, the next morning. The best part of that was, that I was even looking forward to it. Doing something like sport or yoga, followed by a short meditation gave me a feeling of freedom, which accompanied me throughout day. The peaceful start to the morning is worth its weight in gold. Without that, I would have the feeling, that I was missing something.

How did this affect my work? After my 90-minute morning routine, I was filled with fresh inspiration and I was able to start my work efficiently and full of concentration. That way, most of my work was done by midday. I used the evenings for social activities, such as meeting friends and family or taking long walks in the country, instead of working. It felt as if I had much more free time, even though I was doing the same amount of work. In the end, it depends how you organise your day.

Since then I have even moved my daily rhythm forward an hour. I get up at 6am instead of 7am and go to bed an hour earlier. Once I was into the new rhythm, I felt much more like using the extra time in the morning. It is much quieter at 6am and the day looks very different, when it is beginning to dawn. I love this time in the morning to do the things I want to do.

I managed to change from an owl to a lark and do not want to change back to my previous pattern of sleep. The advantages of being a lark, in my opinion, far outweigh the disadvantages. I feel much more relaxed, all day long and more successful than before. I use my 24 hours to its best advantage and get 100% out of my day.

Do you want to achieve that? Then let me inspire you. With motivation and willpower, you too will greet the morning with a smile and contentedly let the day come to a close.

Whether you are a long-sleeper or an early bird, let this book be an inspiration to you, a source of ideas for your evening or morning routine, in order to get the best out of your day.

In this book you will receive background knowledge about sleep and our bodies. This will build the foundation for you to plan your daily routines. In addition, you will receive useful tips on how to improve your morning or evening routines and what you need to be aware of. There are also a few nutrition tips and sport ideas, together with two sets of guidelines to start your day off.

I wish you much success and staying power, in order to achieve your goals in your own personal early bird challenge.

- Chapter 1 -

THE INTERNAL CLOCK

Scientists mostly speak of an internal clock. However, in reality, the body possesses many millions of them. Every single cell has its own timer and every organ has a whole host of them. These clocks are in constant contact with each other in order to maintain the body's rhythm.

I will show you in the next chapter how it works and what goes into it.

DER CIRCADIAN RHYTHM

The circadian rhythm controls the physiological processes of the body in a 24-hour cycle. Within this falls the sleep-wake phases and time orientation together with countless regular and repeating processes, such as sleeping, eating and reproduction. It is called the internal clock and has to adjust itself constantly, due to changing daytime lengths and seasonal changes. These days, we also tend to unbalance our circadian rhythm due to geographical or other changes, such as long-haul flights or working shifts. We notice the results of these changes when our body tries to adjust, causing the so-called jet lag symptoms, such as hunger or sleepiness, which persist until our body has adjusted to the external changes.

These adjustments are prompted by cells in our eyes, called photoreceptors, which are found in the retina. The light information received by these cells are transmitted to the brain. The suprachiasmatic nucleus (SCN) is a part of the hypothalamus and is considered to be the central switching point of the brain. The SCN also coordinates body functions such as:

- Body temperature
- Hormone release
- Variations in blood pressure
- Heart frequency
- Urine production

SLEEP-WAKE RHYTHM

The most important function, which is controlled by the circadian rhythm, is the sleep-wake rhythm. It controls the periodic change between sleeping and waking/consciousness.

Plants also possess a sleep-wake rhythm. As the sun rises in the morning, they open their blossoms and face towards the sun, because they need the sunlight for their metabolism. In the evening, they close their blossoms and the metabolic processes slow down overnight. The next morning, the rhythm starts again from the beginning.

With animals, the sleep-wake rhythm is adapted to the rhythms of the animals they prey on. Nocturnal animals sleep during the day and hunt in the dark. Animals, such as lions, sleep and rest mostly in the hot midday sun and hunt during the cooler morning or evening hours.

WHAT HAPPENS IN THE BODY?

The sleep-wake rhythm is controlled by hormones and the so-called neurotransmitters (chemical messengers in our bodies, which are the connective points between the nerve cells and, from there, they distribute electrical impulses).

Two hormones are prominent in the sleep-wake rhythm: Serotonin and Melatonin.

During the daylight hours, the body produces Serotonin and, at night, production of Melatonin takes over. The production of both substances is strongly dependent on its counterpart.

Serotonin is regarded as the body's own anti-depressive and is therefore known as the "happy hormone". It has a relaxing effect on the body and improves mood, while at the same time being pain-relieving and anti-depressive in nature.

The hormone Melatonin is known as the sleeping hormone. It regulates sleep and is responsible for the rhythm of the hormone cycle. The production of Melatonin is dependent upon the light falling on the retina of the eye. In the dark, when there is no more light available, the production of Melatonin increases, which helps us go to sleep and regulates our sleep phases.

Should the concentration of Melatonin become unbalanced, there is an increase in lethargy, exhaustion and tiredness. Darkness is an important condition for the release of Melatonin. Light reduces the production of Melatonin, which negatively affects the quality of sleep.

In autumn or winter, when there is less light, it can lead to the body having an excess of Melatonin. In the darker seasons, we are missing the light, which is important to keep us fit and well-balanced.

EXTERNAL INFLUENCES

In humans, the sleep-wake rhythm is influenced by, for example, working times. On our free days, our sleep-wake rhythm is usually different to that of the working days.

The body can adjust and get used to the different sleep phases, but mostly the time we wake up is not in sync with the time we should be awake, which causes interference to some of our sleep phases. It can lead to sleeping problems, if the disruption affects certain sleep phases.

DYSFUNCTIONS

You can recognise problems in the function of the sleep-wake rhythm through tiredness, fatigue, exhaustion and increased susceptibility to infections.

If the sleep-wake rhythm is disrupted long-term, depression or psychosis can develop. You can see this best in people suffering from sleep deprivation. After 2-3 nights of sleep deprivation, physical symptoms start to occur, which, if the deprivation continues, can lead to death.

A FEELING FOR TIME

Sometimes time seems to stand still and at other times it seems to run away from us. During meditation some people are able to place themselves in a situation without time or space. Victims of accidents have often stated that they felt the time during the accident as being unnaturally slow. Some people even see their whole life pass before their eyes in one moment. Everyone has experienced, that time, which passes while we are waiting for something to happen, feels like it is taking an age. On the other hand, while reading an interesting book, 30 minutes can seem to fly by extreme quickly.

In everyday life, our days seem to be getting shorter and shorter, because we are so busy. We feel the necessity to pack more and more into the time we have available. We notice it very often at work. A study, written by the German Bundesanstalt für Arbeitsschutz (Federal Institute for Occupational Safety) shows that every second person in Germany is working under great time pressure and more than half of those are suffering because of it.

For decades, scientists have been trying to understand how humans experience time. Experiments, where civilised people return to cave-life, show that we have an automatic clock in our bodies.

In reality, our natural body block does not run in a 24-hour cycle, but a 25-hour cycle. This was discovered by a German psychologist, Jürgen Aschoff, at the beginning of the 1960s, who observed test subjects, who were locked in a bunker without light. The explanation as to why we allow our rhythm to be one hour shorter is probably the sun. Sunlight ensures that our inner clock is synchronised with the 24-hour rhythm of the earth's rotation.

At the same time, the French geologist, Michel Siffre, carried out a similar experiment on himself. He entered a pitch-dark cave in the southern Alps, without a clock, and lived there alone, underground, for two months. He, too, wanted to find out, what effect continual darkness and boredom had on the experience of time and rhythm of the body. He quickly lost his feeling for time and time seemed to pass excruciatingly slowly. Despite that, Siffre's inner clock did not become unbalanced. Even though he lived without sunlight and did not have a clock, he continued a rhythm of slightly more than 24 hours. He slept about 8 hours and was awake for about 16 hours, then became tired.

These experiments brought to light that the body has not one, but two inner clocks. One controls the sleep-wake rhythm and the other is responsible for the feeling of time. Later experiments showed, that these clocks were different, not only in their precision, but also in the times that they measured and were completely independent from external stimulation and consciousness.

This showed, that our body is capable of maintaining the sleep-wake rhythm, even where there is no daylight. Our inner clock tells us, when we are tired or hungry, it regulates heart frequency, metabolism, hormone levels, body temperature and even mental performance. Its own frequency suggests a rhythm of more than a day but it is calibrated to 24 hours.

Something, that the circadian rhythm cannot influence, is the perception of seconds, minutes or hours, that we experience while standing at a traffic light, sitting in the doctor's surgery or waiting for a friend. Researchers call this "interval timing" of the brain; the loss of the concept of time – which Aschoff felt in the bunker and Michel Siffre in the cave – which did not match up with the timing of the circadian rhythm.

LIVING OUT OF STEP WITH THE BIOLOGICAL RHYTHM

If you have to live out of step with your inner clock or find yourself in a situation, where you have no choice but to do so, this could cause psychological and physical problems. If you have to work permanent nights, you are always working against your inner clock. Your body will never completely get used to that, because it is embedded in our genes that our need for sleep is influenced by daylight.

Shift workers, such as doctors or carers, whose work alternates between day and night, fall into a kind of chronic jet-lag effect. This also happens to many people, who go out at weekends, allowing the night to become day, while during the week, they go about their normal rhythm. These people also experience a sort of jet-lag effect at the beginning of the week, just as shift workers do. Then there are additional influencing factors, such as alcohol consumption.

Teachers and lecturers notice, that pupils or students lack concentration or are tired after the weekend because they, too, are suffering from a sort of jet-lag effect.

The annual change from wintertime to summertime also causes many people to feel the consequences. The body must first adjust to the loss or gain of an hour and find its equilibrium again.

- Chapter 2 -

SLEEP

Sometimes we find having to sleep annoying, especially if the late film on the TV is so exciting. We find it difficult to switch off the TV and go to bed. On the other hand, there is nothing nicer than sleeping-in in the mornings. We think staying asleep at this moment would be the most wonderful thing in the world.

However, when we close our eyes, we are on "stand by" and get up a few hours later in this frame of mind. Sleep is a complex procedure, consisting of various phases and cycles. During the night, many important processes take place in our bodies, which help us to stay healthy.

Bearing in mind, that we spend about a third of our lives sleeping, it is worth taking a closer look at what happens when we sleep.

If we want to change our sleeping habits, we first need to understand what happens, in order to optimise it, so that we are refreshed and productive the next morning.

WHY DO WE SLEEP?

A sleeping person looks quiet and peaceful. It is difficult to believe, that many complex processes are taking place during that time.

For a long time, researchers believed, that sleep did not have an important function and was considered to be a "death-like" peace. It was known colloquially as "the little brother of death". Even today, it is not completely understood why humans and animals sleep. However, it is generally accepted, that people need to have enough sleep, in order for them to develop and stay healthy.

PROCESSING INFORMATION

The brain is not in idle mode during sleep. Sleep and brain researchers believe, that the brain is working hard during the night to process the information gained during the day.

Humans are confronted with innumerable stimuli and much information during the day, which has been obtained through the eyes and brain. It seems, we are only aware of a fraction of that. For example, while you are reading these lines, perhaps you are thinking, that you are focused on this book, but at the same time you are absorbing much more information. For example, the light in your environment, sounds or smells. The brain screens out most of that information, because it is considered to be unimportant. Otherwise your brain would not be able to concentrate on reading.

At night, the brain decides which impressions gained during the day should go into the long-term memory and which should be forgotten. The brain's activity can be measured using modern visual procedures and using a brainwave recorder (EEC). These procedures also have the ability of seeing, which parts of the brain are particularly active during the night.

REGENERATION OF THE CARDIO-VASCULAR SYSTEM

Sleep protects us from strokes and diseases of the cardio-vascular system. Shortly after falling asleep, the blood pressure sinks, the pulse slows down to about 50 bpm (a normal adult pulse, while awake and rested, can be anything between 60 and 80 bpm). This is particularly noticeable in the deep sleep phases. The reduced number of beats per minute enables the heart and vascular system to rest. This regeneration is important for the body and reduces the risk of heart attacks and strokes. A study of more than 1,200 participants, carried out by a Japanese scientist, showed, that the risk of such conditions developing sinks dramatically when maintaining a sleep of at least 7.5 hours per night, in comparison to having less sleep.

REGULATING THE METABOLISM

During the day, the body collects metabolic products, which the body purges at night. If you get too little sleep, these products cannot be completely purged, which can cause the metabolism to be out of balance. This leads to an increased risk of contracting "civilisation" conditions, such as diabetes or obesity.

STRENGTHENING THE IMMUNE SYSTEM

During the night, the immune system is very active. It is fighting pathogens and reduces inflammatory processes. This activity reaches its peak in the deep sleep phase. This means, it is possible for a person to sleep himself healthy. This is particularly the case with fever, because sleeping allows the fever to sink. A person can regenerate best during sleep.

In contrast, sleep deprivation can weaken the immune system. There are many studies which prove this. Even short-term sleep deprivation can lead to a significant weakening of the immune system, a statement borne out by Jan Born, a researcher from Lübeck, Germany. For his experiments, he immunised a number of people against Hepatitis A. Half of those immunised were allowed to sleep immediately after the test and the other half had to stay awake until the following evening. Four weeks after the immunisations, blood tests showed, that the half, which had slept after the immunisation, had twice as many antibodies in their blood than those, who had stayed awake. This is a significant effect after even one night of not sleeping.

RELEASE OF GROWN HORMONES

Children mostly grow during sleep. The reason for that is, that a significantly increased amount of growth hormones is produced during the night. These also help to accelerate the healing of wounds, enabling the tissue to regenerate quickly during the night.

Sleep phases, which are too short, lead to the body not being able to regenerate sufficiently. This manifests itself in the morning, after a short night, through wrinkly and impure skin. There is a similar internal effect. It is not immediately noticeable, but it does damage the organs and we age more quickly.

RESTING THE MIND

It is not only the body, which needs rest, sleep also does your mind good. Studies have shown, that people with chronic sleep problems suffer from depression more often than those, who have healthy sleep. This is believed to be due to the fact, that the brain is also able to reorganise itself during sleep, so that it is fresh and ready for the new day. Through sleep, psychological as well as physical health is facilitated.

THE 5 PHASES OF SLEEP

During healthy sleep without disturbances, there are five sleeping phases, which follow in sequence. A whole cycle of five phases takes approximately 90 minutes (for some it is a few minutes more and for some it is a few minutes less). After that, the cycle begins again. This process repeats itself several times during the night. The depth of sleep varies, depending on the individual phase, and it also regulates the amount of rest achieved.

1ST SLEEP PHASE: FALLING ASLEEP (NON-REM PHASE)

As the name suggests, this is the time when we are falling asleep and includes the few minutes after that. During this phase, the body relaxes until we slowly slip off into sleep. The brain goes into a calm mode and the muscle tone decreases – our bodies become limper. Sometimes people experience a feeling of falling or sudden muscle movements in their legs. This happens, when the brain has settled quicker than the body does.

During this phase, the sleep is very light and superficial. The smallest occurrence, such as light or sound can lead to a disturbance in this phase and we wake up again.

2ND SLEEP PHASE: LIGHT SLEEP PHASE (NON-REM PHASE)

After falling asleep, the body goes into a light sleep phase. It sinks deeper into a state of rest. The pulse slows down and our breathing becomes deeper and more relaxed. The body temperature reduces slightly.

The light sleep phase takes up about 30 to 60 minutes of our 90-minute sleep cycle. We find ourselves at least half way through our sleep cycle during this time.

In this phase we begin to process what we have experienced during the day. Our sleep is still superficial and susceptible to disturbances, which cause us to wake up quickly.

3RD AND 4TH SLEEP PHASE: THE DEEP SLEEP PHASE (NON-REM PHASE)

From the light sleep phase, we sink slowly into the deep sleep phase. This is the most regenerative phase for the body and the mind and therefore becomes the most important part of our sleep pattern. It has the most significant influence on the restfulness of our sleep and on the processes within the body.

The deep sleep phase is officially divided into two phases:

- The mid-depth sleep phase
- The very-deep sleep phase

During the deep sleep phase of sleep, as the name suggests, we sleep particularly deeply. At this time, it is particularly hard to wake up. If we are awoken, we initially feel disorientated and groggy and it takes us a while to recover our consciousness.

Sleep-walking or talking in your sleep can happen. This is the time when the body is at its most relaxed. Breathing is peaceful and rhythmical; our muscles and brain activity are run down to the minimum. Our body is on a kind of "stand-by". The pulse and body temperature are at their lowest.

5TH SLEEP PHASE: THE DREAM SLEEP – DIE REM PHASE

After the deep sleep phase, we slip into a short light sleep phase, which leads into the so-called dream phase (also known as the REM phase).

REM means "rapid eye movement" and describes the characteristic quick eye movements behind the closed lids of the eyes, seen during this phase. If you observe these quick eye movements of the eyelids, you know the person is in the REM phase.

It is called the dream phase, because we dream during the REM phase. We also dream during other sleep phases, but during this time, we dream particularly intensive and long. The sleep is significantly lighter during the dream phase and it is easier to be awoken at this time. Sleep researchers assume, that not only information is processed, but also emotional and sense impressions.

The muscles are completely relaxed and almost completely still during the REM phase. It is a kind of natural protection for our bodies, so that we do not carry out the movements, which we are dreaming as this could cause injury.

During the dream phase, our brain frequency intensifies significantly and our pulse increases. We no longer breathe slowly and deeply but more quickly and flatter.

While the deep sleep phase seems to be responsible for the regeneration of the body, the REM sleep seems to be responsible for the necessary psychological recovery.

An adult spends about 20% of his sleeping time in this state. For babies and toddlers, it is significantly more.

SLEEPING CYCLES

These 5 sleep phases repeat themselves about 4 to 7 times per night, depending on the length of time of sleep. This can be illustrated as a kind of sleep cycle staircase: From the falling asleep phase we first go to the light sleep, then deeper into the deep sleep phase, then into the lighter REM sleep, then we arrive back at the light sleep phase.

The first sleep cycle at the beginning of the night shows a particularly long deep sleep phase, which can last up to an hour. The REM phase is comparatively short at about a minute.

During the night, the ratio changes. The deep sleep phase decreases from cycle to cycle and the REM phase increases evermore until the morning. Already, by the third sleep cycle there is a great reduction in the amount of deep sleep, but much longer REM phase sleep. This underlines once more the importance of getting enough sleep at night.

Seen over the whole sleeping length, and in particularly divided over all the sleeping cycles, we find the following ratio per sleep phase:

- Falling asleep phase: 4 - 6%
- Light sleep phase: 45 - 55%
- Mid-depth sleep phase: 4 – 6%
- Deep sleep phase: 12 – 15%
- REM sleep/Dream sleep: 20 – 25%

WAKING UP AT NIGHT

"Sleeping through" does not mean, that we do not wake up at night. On the contrary, good sleep is characterised by several short wake phases. It is possible, that we can wake for a few seconds up to 10 times an hour. During the whole sleep cycle, we could wake up to 23 times, being awake for up to 1 minute.

You do not think it happens to you? That is because you cannot remember it, if the wake time is less than 5 minutes. We only become conscious of it after that period of time. It usually happens 3 to 4 times a night. If it happens more often, and over a longer period of time, we describe our sleep as "disturbed".

In the second half of the night, which is characterised by fewer deep sleep phases, it is possible, that we often wake up for a short time and we recognise that, together with the light sleep in between, as "sleeping through". People, who do not sleep well, remember being awake during these periods, which, in turn, strengthens their fears of not being able to sleep, effectively, leading them to experience even longer wake phases.

Scientists assume, that the reason for these frequent, short periods, when we wake up, is genetic. If we think about the environment, that our ancestors slept in, they were not as safe as today and it is believed, that this short waking up period had a protective function; the need to check the area every now and then in order to guard against possible danger.

By the way, the waking and sleeping phases of a mother adapt to fit with a baby's, as long as they sleep together in one bed. Subconsciously, the mother checks, that her child is safe and changes her position, without remembering it. This is also behaviour, which originates from our ancestors, but even today is very useful.

LENGTH OF SLEEP

Current data shows, that the ideal length of sleep for humans is somewhere between 7 and 8 hours. This is the result of a large-scale study, during which 10,000 test persons were studied for one year. The test subjects had to carry out certain tests during the course of the experiment. The people, who had the worst results, were those, who had slept for less than four hours.

Those, who sleep for less than 6 hours, are known as short-sleepers. Those, who sleep for more than 9 hours, are considered long-sleepers. It is assumed, that short-sleepers sleep more effectively. Although the deep-sleep phases of both types were the same length, it seems, that the long-sleepers' sleep was lighter on average and they dreamed more. This shows, that the length of sleep is not the only important thing to consider. The regenerative value of the sleep is much more important.

Our need for sleep changes during the course of a lifetime, and reduces continuously. After birth, babies sleep an average of 20 hours per day, compared to older people, who often only need 5 hours of sleep.

SLEEP DEFICIT

After a short night, you will notice a reduction in cognitive ability. If we continue to have too little sleep over several days, this can have serious effects. It is the equivalent of having a blood alcohol content of 0.6.

It was seen on test persons, that after chronic sleep deprivation, they perceived themselves to be fitter and more awake than they were in reality. The loss of performance, through sleep deficit and its consequences, is often underestimated.

ORIGINS OF SLEEP DEFICIT

There are many different reasons why people get too little sleep. When people, whether for business or private reasons, pass through several time zones, they often suffer from jet lag. This includes those, who are permanently travelling, such as pilots or flight attendants.

Other occupational groups, such as shift workers or night workers, working in hospitals or in security, also suffer from mild jet lag symptoms or sleep deficit after working on changing shifts for months. This occupational group covers 16% of all employees. They are particularly vulnerable to making mistakes because of sleep deficit. Sleeping against your circadian rhythm shortens the length of your sleep on the one side, and impairs the quality of your sleep on the other. A large proportion of people within this occupational group complain of sleep disturbances and resort to self-therapy, such as caffeine, nicotine or alcohol.

In addition to the at-risk occupational groups, in our society, we are all subject to increased risk of chronic sleep deficit. This is partly due to our lifestyle. We all have multiple obligations, working the whole day and after that, having to go shopping and do other things. After watching TV in the evening, relaxing or meeting friends, you look at the clock and, suddenly, it is already so late and you have not finished everything yet.

Working hours are fixed in most occupations due to social constraints. When we are busy with many things and do not get to bed in time, the alarm clock still rings at the usual time, even if we have not had enough sleep.

Till Roenneberg of the Ludwig-Maximilian University, Munich, and his team analysed data from 65,000 Europeans. They determined, that the average sleeping time of those between 40 and 55 years during working days was regularly less than 7 hours. Proof, that this was not enough, was shown by the results of the weekend sleeping patterns of those people, which showed, that they slept longer at the weekends, on average by one hour. Pre-school children and pensioners were different. Results showed even sleeping times for this group during week days and weekends. The cause of the sleep deficit of the first group was called by researchers the "social jet lag", because the biological sleeping rhythm did not fit with the normal, socially-accepted sleep-wake rhythm.

CONSEQUENCES

Apart from the gruelling daytime tiredness, people with sleep deficit often suffer other dangerous effects:

Danger of Diabetes:

Too little sleep changes the regulation of the blood sugar. The glucose tolerance and sensitivity for Insulin sink. Both are seen as the precursor for Diabetes Type 2. Other studies show, that sleep deficit upsets the hormone saturation regulation. It tends to secrete the appetite-stimulating hormone Ghrelin. Tiredness also makes you hungry and you eat more than you would do, if you had slept enough. This, in turn, influences the blood glucose level.

Higher Susceptibility to Infection:

Sufficient sleep is very important in achieving a strong immune system. Too little sleep, however, subdues the immune system and the body becomes more susceptible to infections. In 2015, the Californian neuroimmunologist, Aric Prather, and his team, subjected test persons to a head-cold-inducing virus (Rhinovirus), using a spray. The result was: The test subjects, who had slept for less than six hours during the previous two weeks, were 4 times more likely to catch the virus than those, who had slept normally.

<u>Danger of having accidents and making mistakes:</u>
Too little sleep leads to concentration and memory disorders and slows down reaction time. It can also cause short breaks in awareness or attention or even lead to microsleep. This is particularly dangerous, when driving a vehicle. Countless accidents occur each year because of sleep deficit and microsleeping.

8 TIPS FOR BETTER SLEEP

1. *Sleeping environment:*

Optimum design of the bedroom and bed can work wonders. A bedside lamp with cosy, dim lighting, for example, can put you in a comfortable evening mood. Having nice bedcovers, various pillows and a nice picture on the wall can add to the pleasant atmosphere, so that you feel comfortable in your bedroom and enjoy going to bed.

The ideal temperature for sleeping is somewhere between 17 and 22 degrees centigrade (approximately 63°-72°F). We often make the mistake of having the bedroom temperature too high, particularly in winter. This causes the air to dry out. During the winter, a humidifier could help to ease the situation.

2. *Keep your sleeping rhythm:*

A regular sleep-wake rhythm is very important for good sleep quality. The effectiveness is increased by having a consistent evening and morning routine. Our inner clock shows us, that we naturally get tired in the evening and wake up refreshed, as long as we do not disturb our sleep-wake rhythm. Try to keep to the same routine at the weekends.

3. *Sport:*

Doing sport during the day helps to enable good sleep. You should avoid doing strenuous training shortly before bed, because this activates the circulation of your body. You would feel stimulated and probably would not be able to go straight off to sleep. The body needs some time to settle down.

Light physical activities, such as a one-hour walk in the afternoon or early evening, can help you to sleep better.

4. *Lighter meals:*

It is not recommended to eat large meals just before going to bed. Having a full stomach is not good for sound sleep, because the body is busy digesting the food, that is already there. Try to arrange your evenings so, that you do not eat anything later than 2 hours before going to bed, or if you do, only something light.

5. *Avoid caffeine, alcohol and nicotine:*

You should avoid caffeine from the afternoon onwards. It can take up to 5 hours for even half the caffeine to work its way out of your body. Caffeine causes difficulties when trying to go off to sleep. This causes you to sleep lighter and shorter.

Alcohol makes you tired and lets you go to sleep faster, but that does not mean, that you sleep better. Regular consumption of alcohol can, in the long term, lead to sleeping disorders.

Nicotine keeps you awake. Even hours after you have smoked your last cigarette, it disrupts the quality of your sleep. Almost every third smoker does not sleep well, because the nicotine levels of their body sink during the night.

6. *Meditation, breathing and relaxation exercises:*

Scientific studies show, that slow, controlled breathing sinks the heartrate and blood pressure, which in turn settles the whole body. Suitable methods to achieve that include meditation and relaxation techniques, such as autogenic training and Jacobson's progressive muscle relaxation.

7. *Relaxing music:*

I recommend quiet, classical music to help you to go to sleep. The music should come to a stop slowly and gently, in order to avoid an abrupt end, which would wake you up again.

8. *Avoid blue light:*

Probably the most important point, and at the same time most difficult, is the avoidance of blue light from your laptop, tablet or smartphone. Those, who sit for a long time in front of an LED screen, are said to be delaying their sleep-wake rhythm, according to the Swiss sleep researcher, Christian Cajochen. The blue wavelengths of this light made of Light-Emitting Diodes (LED), which illuminate your mobile phone or laptop, make us alert and adversely affect the regulation of the hormones, which are responsible for our sleep.

Try to avoid using your mobile phone or laptop two hours before going to bed, or if you do, use the blue-light filter, which a lot of modern devices possess.

- Chapter 3 -

OWLS AND LARKS

Are you one of those people, who are wide awake early in the morning and always get up full of the joys of spring? Or do you prefer to sleep longer because you do not get tired until late in the evening? Long-sleepers and early birds are a natural phenomenon. The sleep-wake rhythm of most people is somewhere between the morning-fresh lark and the night-active owl.

Scientists have named both extremes of the sleep-wake rhythm after birds. Larks are active in the early morning, whereas owls are not active until the night-time.

LARKS: EARLY BIRDS

You often find, that managers are larks. They are up early in the morning and are going about their jobs before others are awake.

- Apple CEO Tim Cook: He is known as a real early bird. It is said, that he wakes up at 3:45 am to do his emails and so that there is enough time for him to train in his fitness studio before he goes to work.

- Claus Hipp, Chief of the Hipp baby food producers: He wakes up at 4:30 am. Before he goes to work, he visits his chapel for his morning contemplation.

- Twitter founder Jack Dorsey: His day starts a little later but even so he is up at 5:30 am. Before his day's work begins, he meditates or jogs 10 miles.

Working hours in our society favour the larks. The early daily routine is completely compatible with the timing of the bio-rhythm. The performance of the early bird is positively influenced by the fact, that those, who are at work early, being the first in the office, are less likely to be inundated with phone calls or disturbed by colleagues.

In everyday working life, larks are much more at an advantage, compared to owls. Larks find more difficulty in fitting in a social life, which often takes place in the evenings, after everyone is finished at work. Typical larks, who get out of bed early, become tired earlier. Because of this, larks tend not to participate as much in evening activities.

OWLS: LATE RISERS

There are also many successful people among the late risers. Here are some of them:

- Amazon CEO, Jeff Bezos: He is considered to be the richest man in the world. He makes sure, that he gets 8 hours sleep each night. "For me, that is the necessary amount to have enough energy", he said in an interview.

- Microsoft founder, Bill Gates: As an owl, he often goes to bed at midnight and allows himself 7 hours sleep. He needs that, he says, to be sharp, creative and to stay in a good mood.

- Albert Einstein, the brilliant physicist: He liked to stay in bed for up to 10 hours. Significant thoughts about the theory of relativity came to him in his sleep.

It is considerably more difficult for owls to reconcile their biorhythm with external factors. They are wide awake in the evenings and then, if they are awoken early in the morning, they suffer mostly from sleep deficit. This constant stress can have a negative long-term effect on the owl.

WHO IS MORE SUCCESSFUL?

There appear to be successful people among the owls and the larks. Which type, then, is more successful? There have been countless studies on this subject and it seems to be a question, which occupies many people. Here is a small selection of the facts, which have been proven by studies.

1. In a study with students, the biologist, Prof. Christoph Randler determined, that early birds are more successful. Early risers win by a nose when it comes to success. They tend to achieve better results at school, which leads them to attending better universities, which, in turn, improves their career chances. In addition, they are said to be better at predicting problems and are more proactive, he said in an interview. Many studies have confirmed a connection between proactivity, better work performance, success in their job and higher wages.

2. The Belgian doctor, Dr. Philippe Peigneux, proved, using brain scanners, that night owls become quicker workers than larks, 10.5 hours after getting up, when they are less sleepy. However, the results 1.5 hours after getting up were similar in both groups.

3. A current long-term study from Britain involving 430,000 people between the ages of 38 and 73 shows, that owls have a greater risk of developing diabetes, respiratory and gastrointestinal disorders. In addition, they die younger than early birds. Various possible reasons for this are speculated: Stress, sleep deficit and an unhealthy diet.

4. An experiment with students at the Harvard University was carried out where they had to remember 100 words, recounting as many of them as they could 12 hours later. Half the students were given the words at 9am and the other half were given their words in the evening, so that

they could sleep on them. The result was: The sleep-refreshed students could remember many more of these words than the others, showing that long-sleepers can process much more information in their subconscious minds.

5. A study by Christopher M. Barnes, an American university professor, showed, that if a company offers flexible working hours, the manager evaluated the workers, who come to work early better than those, who come later. This even applied, if the performance of both workers was similarly good.

6. Psychologists of the University of Milan determined, that of the 120 participants tested, the owls were more creative than the larks. The participants had to solve various tasks where the mental flexibility and richness of ideas of an artistic work was evaluated. Owls have to improvise in their jobs a lot, particularly in the mornings, because of their daily rhythm. It

can be assumed, that this is the reason why their creativity is better trained.

7. Franzis Preckel, a highly-talented researcher from the University of Trier, was able to determine, by gathering data from various studies, that there is a slight positive correlation between evening activity and intelligence. Early birds, however, showed better academic performance. Her conclusions from this study: Those, who are active longer in the evenings, and have to get up early in the mornings, are less likely to be able to achieve their full potential in performance, because of their sleep deficit.

In conclusion, it can be said, that both types have their strengths. The owls have, however, significantly more difficulty in today's society if they are not able to work the hours, which suit them. A lark is able to plan much more effectively and get more out of the day.

SELF TEST

Are you a natural owl or lark? People are not necessarily one or the other. There are also mixtures of both. In addition, people change their sleeping type during their lives. If you are an owl, it does not mean that you will always be an owl.

The test is designed to determine, who belongs in which group. It can be very interesting to repeat the test, just after ending the early riser challenge and compare it to the first result. Have your sleeping habits and daily activities changed as a result of the challenge, or have they remained the same?

THE TEST
1. *When do you normally go to bed?*
   - I go to bed mostly before 10pm and go to sleep quickly. (1 point)
   - Mostly, I go to bed between 10pm and 1am. (3 points)
   - I never go to bed at the same time. (2 points)

2. *How well do you sleep through?*
   - I keep waking up early in the morning. (2 points)
   - I nearly always sleep right through. (1 point)
   - I have trouble going to sleep, but then I mostly sleep right through. (3 points)

3. *How do you wake up?*
   - I like to snooze in the morning. I do not like getting up. (3 points)
   - I am often awake before the alarm goes off and I get straight up. (1 point)

- I wake up at a different time every day. (2 points)

4. *How do you feel in the morning?*
   - I am awake and fit directly after getting up. (1 point)
   - It depends how quickly I wake up. (2 points)
   - I need a lot of time in the morning until I am properly awake. (3 points)

5. *At which time during the day do you feel most effective?*
   - I am at my most effective in the morning or early afternoon. (1 point)
   - My best performance is varied, depending on the day. (2 points)
   - I am at my best in the afternoons or evenings. (3 points)

6. *When do you usually plan to do important tasks?*
   - I often plan my day spontaneously. (2 points)

- I plan to do important things in the evening. (3 points)
- I try to carry out important tasks in the morning. (1 point)

7. *When do you regenerate best?*
   - Night-time is the best time for me to relax. (3 points)
   - I cannot relax and switch off properly until the evenings. (1 point)
   - I relax at different times during the day. (2 points)

8. *When do you wake up on your free days?*
   - I wake up early, even if I am off work. (1 point)
   - I like to sleep in. (3 points)
   - If I am off work, sometimes I wake up earlier, sometimes later. (2 points)

SCORES

Add all the points of your answers together and compare the number to the table below to find out which sleeping type you are:

8 to 12 Points: Lark

You are an early bird by nature. You prefer to work and carry out important tasks in the mornings. Perhaps you are not yet using your biorhythm properly. Now is the time to optimise your morning routine to utilise your potential, as an early bird to its best advantage.

13 to 18 Points: Mixed type

You are a mixed type. It is not clear whether you are a lark or an owl. You are more the sort of person, who varies their sleeping habits. Sometimes you find it easy to get up and sometimes you would rather stay up all night. Changing to a regular sleep-wake rhythm could help you to go to sleep and wake up more easily.

19 to 24 Points: Owl

You are definitely an owl. The morning is not particularly your friend and waking up is a daily fight. You probably belong to the people, who like to use the snooze option on your alarm and like to stay in bed a few minutes longer, until you really have to get up to go to work. For you it would be significantly more difficult to change your sleep-wake rhythm, than it would be for another sleeping type. The good news is, that it is also not impossible for you, as long as you have the necessary motivation.

- Chapter 4 -

MORNING ROUTINE

Most people do not really have a set morning routine. Drinking your coffee and then leaving the house for work is part of that. The morning routine is a personal, conscious routine, designed to organise the first hours of the day, and which will become a habit.

To make your morning routine helpful to you, it should be:

- Chosen by yourself
- Incorporating your aims
- Carried out daily
- Bring positive effects
- Reconciled to your personal needs
- Seen as a long-term commitment.

The customisation of your routine to your personal needs plays a big role in this. It should do you good and you should experience positive effects in the long-term.

Take, for example, doing a yoga exercise after getting up: On the one hand it is something, that you like to do and you notice, that the back pains, which you get from sitting all day, have started to improve. If that is the case, it is easier for you to incorporate that into your morning routine than something, which does not motivate you as much, for example, jogging. During the first few days it would probably be difficult for you to get up early and go jogging. After that, you would probably do it less and less until you stop doing it altogether. It is different with things, which you prefer to do and which you enjoy.

The aim of the morning routine is, that it happens continually, i.e. every day. If not, it becomes a morning activity, but not a routine. It does not have to take hours; most people do not have that much time. You should plan your morning routine according to the time you have available and how much of it you want to spend on your routine.

REASONS WHY IT IS WORTH USING THOSE EARLY MORNING HOURS.

If you start the day in a bad way, it tends to continue throughout the day. A good morning routine can help you to start your day in a good way.

People are said to be creatures of habit and this is where the morning routine comes into its own. Hectic and stress in the morning quickly become a habit and every day begins in the same uncomfortably way and could even be harmful.

However, if you manage to change those habits and to optimise your morning routine, you will experience many advantages.

Better Performance:
In the morning, our head is still clear and free of impressions and information, which gather during the day. It is easier to concentrate, you become more productive and your performance improves.

More Discipline:

Your willpower is at its highest early in the morning. This helps you to stay disciplined and work towards your own goals. If you start something in the morning, the chances that you will continue it to the end, are greater.

More Focus:

If you are up and about before the others, you have the great advantage, that you can work undisturbed. There are no telephone calls or discussions with colleagues to distract you from your work. You can focus on your own work, without all the interruptions.

More Efficiency:

Because it is quiet in the morning, you are in a better position to achieve more in a shorter time. You can utilise the time to your best advantage. You would be able to do much more than you could, for example, in the afternoon or evening.

More Productivity:

Once you are "in the flow" in the mornings, this will carry on throughout the day and you will be more productive than if you start the day in a sluggish way and try to improve as the day goes on.

More Satisfaction:

When you look back, during your lunch break, to your morning's work, you notice, that you have been very productive. This success produces satisfaction and motivates you to continue in this way. This motivation helps you, ultimately, to carry out your morning routine every day.

THE MOST COMMON MISTAKES IN THE MORNING ROUTINE

The biggest mistake you can make is not to have a morning routine at all. But you are in the process of making positive changes and you are going in the right direction to become a successful early bird.

However, there are some common mistakes, which can be made in the morning routine and should be avoided.

1. *Excuses:*

You need to have a certain measure of discipline with your morning routine. As soon as you start making excuses like: "Today I will sleep a little longer" or "I do not like to go jogging in this weather", the more likely you are to use the excuses and be less consistent. Regarding out-door activities, which are dependent on the weather, I suggest having an alternative, which you can carry out inside, so that your activity does not stop completely.

2. *Distractions:*

In the morning, we tend to dawdle and are easily distracted. During your morning routine, you should concentrate completely on your activity. Do not let yourself be distracted – for example turn off your smartphone resolutely, so as not to be tempted to look at social media – this is how valuable time gets wasted.

3. *Hectic:*

Up to now, you have been starting your day in a hectic way. The aim of the morning routine is to achieve the opposite, to start the day peacefully. If you are stressed in the morning by things you have to do, this does not add up to a good morning routine. Only plan enough things into your routine, which you can carry out with a certain calmness.

4. *Aimlessness:*

Getting up and doing things without a plan does not hold much promise of success, it robs you of the time, which you could put to better use. A morning routine must be planned before it can be successful. Plan your morning routine and follow your objectives in order to achieve your goals.

5. *Imitation:*

Of course, you could follow examples of the morning routines of other people, but this does not stand much chance of success. Those people are only successful with their routines because they chose them themselves. So, it is not such a good idea to copy other people. Find out what you want to plan into your morning, so that it fits your own needs.

6. *Volatility:*

Doing one thing for two days, and the next days doing something else, could be the right thing to do at the beginning to find your best routine, but you need to set what does you good, and what you would like to do every morning, as quickly as possible. Once you have chosen your activities, stick to them and let them become your routine.

7. *Smartphone after waking up:*

We know, that most people go for their smartphones as soon as they wake up. People mostly use the alarm function of their mobile phone, so firstly, the alarm has to be switched off. After that, you open your social media account and look at your WhatsApp messages. This is very common behaviour in today's world of digitalisation.

However, this development is poisonous. The flood of information, which storms the brain within just a few seconds overwhelms us and leads to compulsive behaviour. With every "like" or "share" you receive from your postings and every received message, your brain releases happy hormones and you want more of them. This behaviour is comparable to an alcohol addiction. Today's young generation is shockingly badly affected by this. The so-called smartphone addiction or internet addiction is not yet recognised as such in our society. It is not considered normal behaviour these days to withdraw from media and smartphone consumption.

We often spend more time on social media, than we intended to and that way we lose valuable minutes in the morning, which could have been better utilised with a clear head. In the mornings we are particularly sensitive to the positive stimuli afforded by the smartphone. Many people look at their mobile phone the moment they wake up. The brain is then re-programmed to scatter during the most sensitive phase of waking up and this leads to an addiction in the search for approval through "likes", "shares" or messages.

One of the biggest mistakes in the morning routine is to use the smartphone or internet within the first 3 hours after waking up. This increases the risk of smartphone addiction and destroys the concentration and productivity needed in the coming day.

Avoid the distractions of smartphone and internet in the morning before it becomes a habit and has a negative impact on you.

8. *Snooze Function:*

The snooze function of your alarm causes another problem, particularly because many people use their smartphones, which have the snooze function on them. Very few people these days use the good old radio alarm or even an analogue alarm.

"If I only sleep 5, 10 or 15 minutes longer, then getting up will surely be easier", most people think.

Unfortunately, this is not the case – snoozing is not helpful in getting up. Sleeping a few minutes longer will not make you feel any more rested than getting up directly after the first alarm rings.

While snoozing, the first thoughts start to enter your head, such as "Today will be a tiring day", or "Oh no, today is my performance review" and will inevitably enter your sleepy consciousness.

It is better to avoid the snooze function and the morning ponderance and rather enjoy a clear head in the morning. Try hopping out of bed at the first alarm so that you do not lose so much time before you start your morning routine. A tip: Put your smartphone or alarm clock out of reach so that you have to get up to turn it off. Once you are on your feet, your day can start.

WHAT HELPS YOU TO GET UP IN THE MORNING?

It depends on the person as to what helps them to get up in the mornings. Try to find out what is best for you and what supports you in starting your day full of the joys of spring. Two of the most important points have already been mentioned in the previous chapter: Avoid smartphones and LED monitors, such as that of your laptop early in the morning and forego the "snooze". In addition to those, there are a few more useful tips, such as these:

<u>The Alarm:</u>
The way we wake up in the morning also has a bearing on our whole day. An annoying alarm sound is probably not the best way to wake up, compared to, for example, music helping you gently out of your sleep. The best kind of music is something with a driving beat or energy-packed songs, which invite you to sing and dance. Whether you choose your favourite song or another energetic song is up to you. Some people prefer not to play their favourite song, because they would get fed up with it after a few days. Other

people love to hear their favourite songs to get them into a good mood. You can change your wake-up song regularly, so that you do not spoil your enjoyment of it.

Unfortunately, it is often not possible to wake up with the sunlight. It is usually dark when you wake up early in the morning, for the majority of the year, and pitch black in your bedroom until the sun rises, sometime later. Light alarms could help to imitate the missing sunlight. The bedside lights are set to light up 20 to 60 minutes before the alarm goes off and become increasingly brighter. This releases the body's own happy hormone, Serotonin, and slows down the production of the sleep hormone, Melatonin. Both these effects help you to wake up in a natural and pleasant way.

<u>Smiling:</u>

This is something small with a great effect. Wake up and greet the morning with a smile. This causes the release of numerous happy hormones in the brain and lets you start the day in an enjoyable way. Smile at the morning and it will smile back at you! Try to smile for the first few minutes of every day. You will be surprised what a difference it makes to your body.

Positive Thinking:

Instead of thinking what challenges the day will bring, it is more productive to start the day with positive thoughts. What are you looking forward to the most today? Try to block out what stresses you and keep the good things on your mind. Will you be meeting a friend? Or do you plan to have a nice long walk in the park? Think of what pleasant things you will be doing every day. You should always be able to think of something, because only then can it be a good day.

Fresh Air:

Open the window and let in the fresh air as soon as you wake up. This expels the tiredness and provides the brain with Oxygen. The air in the morning is mostly cool and this helps to lift your spirits and get yourself moving.

Cold Shower:

The feared cold shower in the morning does not seem so inviting at first. That said, it has an enormous effect on our bodies and starts the circulation going, so that you feel fresh and fit. Of course, you do not need to stand under the cold shower for 10 minutes, that is too much to expect, particularly in the colder seasons. Try to have hot/cold sequence showers and you will see, that you will become more resistant to the cold over time.

Early Sport:

Sport is very effective in waking you up in the mornings. You are not the sporty type? It does not matter, 5 – 7 minutes yoga or power training is enough to get your circulation going full swing. Those who cannot do any sport at all in the mornings could give themselves a thorough stretch of all their limbs, directly after getting up. If you are very sporty, try to run once around the block. Early sport has the added advantage of letting you feel good throughout the day. If you do your training unit early in the morning, you will feel fit and alive and will have time in the evening for other things.

Sport before or after breakfast? Short, light training units can be carried out before breakfast. Otherwise I recommend having a light breakfast before your work-out. Everyone has a different metabolism and reacts differently. Find out what suits you best.

Healthy Breakfast:

Most people are used to leaving the house on an empty stomach, perhaps they have time for a quick cup of tea or coffee. Having a light breakfast boosts the metabolism, the body processes get moving and begin to deliver energy for the day. In addition, it provides important vitamins and minerals.

Going to bed in good time

In order to ensure, that you can get up early, of course you need to go to bed earlier than you are perhaps used to doing. You need to find out the right time for yourself. Some only need 6 hours sleep and others need 8 hours. It could be helpful to know your sleep cycle, when planning your bedtime.

- Chapter 5 -

FOOD AND DRINK

The nutrition and beverages, that you consume during the day, have a great influence on your sleep patterns. In order to keep a regular sleep-wake rhythm, it could be worth evaluating your nutrition and perhaps making some changes.

CAFFEINE

For some people, it is difficult to imagine life without caffeine. A cup of coffee in the morning wakes you up and few people want to do without it. The effects of caffeine can be felt about 30 minutes after consumption and last for about 4 hours.

This is how caffeine works in our systems:

- A high dose of caffeine increases the pulse. For those, who only seldom consume caffeine, it can lead to an increase in blood pressure.

- Even small doses of caffeine can improve concentration and stave off tiredness, short-term.

- Caffeine causes narrowing of the blood vessels in the brain. This can lead to a light alleviation of headaches and migraines.

- When we consume caffeine, the muscles receive a better supply of oxygen. This is why a lot of sporty people take caffeine tablets.

Regular consumption of caffeine causes the body to get used to its effects, so that its effectiveness decreases over time.

Too much caffeine consumption can cause headaches, sleep disorders, nervousness, restlessness and gastro-intestinal complaints.

The European authorities for food safety determined that 200 mg caffeine per single dose and 400 mg per day is harmless for the body. With children, the safe level is a maximum of 3 mg caffeine per kilogram of body weight.

The amount of caffeine in a cup of coffee depends on several factors. It depends on whether the coffee is hot or cold roasted and brewed, how long it brews for, which beans are used, and how fine the beans are milled. Guideline values are as below, although they can vary:

- Coffee: 50 mg per 100 ml
- Espresso: 130 mg per 100 ml

- Black and green tea: 20 mg per 100 ml
- Coca-Cola: 10 mg per 100 ml
- Club Mate: 20 mg per 100 ml
- Red Bull: 32 mg per 100 ml
- Dark chocolate: 90 mg per 100 g
- Whole milk chocolate: 15 mg per 100 g

A 250 ml cup of coffee therefore contains about 125 mg of caffeine. A lot of people do not know that chocolate contains caffeine, particularly dark chocolate.

THEANINE OR CAFFEINE IN TEA?

The active ingredient in green and black tea is Theanine. This is also caffeine, but it is bonded onto Polyphenols. The caffeine is not released until it reaches the bowel, which means, that it takes longer for it to take effect, but it also lasts longer.

A cup of green tea can get you through the day with as much power as a cup of coffee. However, the caffeine boost is not as noticeable as it is with coffee, but lasts longer.

Bear in mind, that the effect of the caffeine in green tea reduces over time, if it is left too long to brew. The longer it is left to brew, the more tannin will seep into the water from the leaves, which reacts with the caffeine to block its effect. In addition, the tea could easily become bitter. On the other hand, the green tea does not produce enough effect, if it is not brewed for long enough, because the leaves have not had enough time to release their caffeine. I recommend a brew time of 1 to 2 minutes. This way you will be fit, but the tea will not taste bitter.

ALCOHOL

"A glass of wine before bed and then you will sleep better", a lot of people think so – but they are wrong. Alcohol really does help you initially to go off to sleep, because the alcohol reduces the activity in the brain, thereby reducing the buzz of thoughts passing through. However, getting off to sleep quicker has its price. The quality of your sleep is much worse, if you drink alcohol before going to bed and this can lead to sleep disorders, as many studies have substantiated. Alcohol makes you wake up more often and it can cause more frequent visits to the bathroom. A large amount of alcohol dries the body out, which means, that, after every visit to the bathroom, there is a need to drink water to quench your thirst. You can feel the effects of the alcohol in the morning. You do not feel rested and are tired, making your sleep less regenerative.

Alcohol is an addictive substance. People, who regularly use it to help them sleep, also risk becoming dependent on it. If you want to sleep well and peacefully, please take the following into consideration:

- Generally only drink alcohol in moderation.
- Allow about 4 to 6 hours after your last alcoholic drink before going to bed.

RULES FOR A GOOD BREAKFAST

English-speakers use the term breakfast, meaning "breaking the fast", the French call it petit-déjeuner, which means "Little fast breaking". The German expression "Frühstück" comes from the 15th century, according to the Duden, and means something like "the piece of bread, which is eaten in the early morning". That remains unchanged, the typical German breakfast today includes bread or bread buns.

At the weekends, 87% of Germans wake up to bread or bread buns on the breakfast table. With it you will find butter, jam, cold meats, cheese and eggs. However, more and more people are trying out variations from other countries. Some like the full English breakfast of eggs, bacon and sausage, others prefer the French variation of croissants and white coffee, or latte as it is now known.

For about 37% of Germans, breakfast is the most important meal of the day, during the week, even more so than lunch or dinner.

The following three rules will help you to get started with a good breakfast:

RULE 1: WHOLEGRAIN

Wholegrain is full of dietary fibre. The German corporation for nutrition (DGE) recommends an amount of 30g per day. 2 slices of wholegrain bread (100g) contain 8g of fibre (compared to a kiwi at 75g). This way you can satisfy a third of your daily needs.

According to the DGE, dietary fibre not only keeps you from feeling hungry, but also helps to prevent high blood pressure and coronary heart disease, and probably also reduces the risk of developing diabetes Type 2.

RULE 2: REDUCE SUGAR

Please be aware, that there is a lot of sugar hidden in many products where you would not necessarily expect it. This simple sugar sends your blood glucose level skyrocketing and then sinks as rapidly, and therefore is not conducive to maintaining an optimum energy level.

Sugary foodstuffs, such as crunchy flakes or Nut-Nougat cream contain unnecessary "empty calories", which are better avoided.

RULE 3: REDUCE UNHEALTHY FAT

In addition to sugar, there is often hidden unhealthy fat in food and drinks. For example, in latte macchiato or caffè latte but also in cold meats, such as salami and other processed foods. These saturated fats increase blood lipids, particularly the harmful LDL-cholesterol.

HEALTHY ALTERNATIVES

There are healthy alternatives, which taste just as good and help you to make a healthy start into your day, to provide you with valuable vitamins and deliver optimum energy to the body.

Natural Yoghurt:

Yoghurt contains valuable proteins, calcium and magnesium and is ideal to eat for breakfast. Fruit yoghurt, however, usually contains too much unnecessary sugar – there can be up to four lumps of sugar in one cup.

Natural yoghurt is the low-sugar variant. If you do not want to do without the fruit taste, you can add some fruit puree or shredded apple to it. If you are missing the sweetness, you can add a little honey, maple syrup or date syrup.

By the way, have you ever tried coconut yoghurt? This is the vegan yoghurt alternative, based on coconut milk. It is mild-tasting, sugar-free and suitable for people with lactose or gluten intolerance.

Fruit spreads:

A fruit spread would be a good alternative to nut-nougat cream, as it can help to save some of the sugar and fat content in chocolate spread. If possible, you should make it yourself or at least look at the sugar content when buying it. Bread spreads, such as honey, date syrup or maple syrup are sweet and have many positive characteristics as long as they are natural products. The sweetness is very similar to that of the chocolate spread.

Muesli

Bought crispy muesli mixes often contain a lot of sugar and fats. As an alternative, you can mix your own muesli. These include, for example, oat flakes, chia seeds, sesame, sunflower seeds or goji berries. Add a few spoonsful of natural yoghurt and a few fresh fruits and you have created a balanced and quickly prepared breakfast.

If you allow chia seeds seep in water overnight, you can make them into a sort of pudding. They are very healthy and low in calories. You can also prepare raw oats for your muesli: To do that, you can soak the oats overnight in milk or water to soften them.

Fat-reduced variations

Do you prefer a hearty breakfast? Salami contains a lot of fat, lean ham would be a less fatty solution. Or perhaps you like fish. Smoked salmon is also a healthy option because it contains valuable Omega-3 fatty acids, which we tend to eat too little of in our diets. Omega-3 fatty acids help to sink the LDL-Cholesterol in the blood, have a positive effect on the brain function and are anti-inflammatory.

NUTRITION TIPS FOR HEALTHY SLEEP

What and when we eat and drink has a significant influence on our sleep. Food, which remains heavy in the stomach from dinner, do not help the situation. Using a few tricks, you can improve your sleep.

WHEN TO EAT

Between eating the last meal of the day and going to bed, there should be at least 2 or 3 hours. If you leave too long between eating and going to bed, you could become hungry and that is not helpful when trying to go to sleep.

A gap, which is too short, can lead to you feeling uncomfortably full in bed and is also not conducive to sleep. The golden middle of 2 – 3 hours is the best solution.

A NAP AFTER LUNCH?

The afternoon nap, after a large lunch is a well-established habit in many cultures. Eating makes you tired because the body needs energy for digesting the food. If you need your energy for digestion, it is missing if needed for activities. It can be hard at times going back to work after lunch and many people think, that a small nap would be just the thing. However, sleeping in the afternoon makes it more difficult to sleep at night, if you are not used to it. Lying down after a large meal can also cause heartburn. Many people believe, you should avoid sleeping in the afternoon, although scientific opinions are divided and there is not yet a final evaluation on this.

WHEN AND WHAT TO EAT

The simplest rule of thumb says: The later you eat, the lighter you should eat. Food, which is difficult to digest, disrupts your attempts to go to sleep. Try to avoid food, which causes flatulence, such as wholegrain bread or pulses. Also avoid French fries or pork steaks. I recommend lean foods, such as turkey breast, low-fat milk and not too much seasoning to make a light evening meal.

Milk contains sleep-inducing Tryptophan, as do fish or dates. Vitamin B6 can also have a positive effect on sleep. This can be found in bananas and many types of salad leaves.

WHEN SHOULD I DRINK MY LAST CAFFEINE-CONTAINING BEVERAGE?

Those who have difficulty going off to sleep, should stop drinking caffeine-containing beverages, such as coffee or energy drinks by 4pm at the latest.

Caffeine and guarana, which can be found in many energy drinks, are broken down very slowly in the body. You should avoid drinking something like this at least 4 hours before going to bed.

It is a similar situation with green and black tea. As everybody reacts differently and has different tolerance levels, it pays to experiment to find out when it is the right time to stop drinking caffeine-containing beverages, so that you can go off to sleep.

WHICH TEAS/HERBAL INFUSIONS INDUCE SLEEP?

Herbal infusions are particularly good to drink at night, because they have relaxing and sleep-inducing qualities. You do not have to drink the same sort of herbal infusion every evening. You can vary it and this way you can also find out, which one is best for helping you sleep.

The following infusions are recommended:

- Valerian
- Melissa
- Camomile
- Passion flower
- Lemon balm
- Magnolia
- Lavender
- St. John's wort
- Catnip

IS A BEDTIME SWEET ALLOWED?

From the sleep scientist's and doctor's points of view, something sweet at bedtime is allowed and can even have a positive effect. A little milk chocolate, a cup of warm cocoa, a few biscuits or a portion of sweet fruit influences the blood glucose level, so that you can sleep better. A small amount of something sweet is also soothing and you are not in danger of dependency on it, nor does it disturb the quality of your sleep as alcohol would do. Just do not forget to clean your teeth afterwards and only eat a little!

- Chapter 6 -

ACTIVATING BODY AND MIND

Sport and relaxation techniques have been scientifically proved to have a positive effect on your sleep-wake rhythm. Your body always needs a balanced amount of activity and quiet.

EARLY MORNING SPORT

Admittedly, most people are not really up to doing sport, shortly after waking up. During the first minutes of being awake, you are not yet feeling refreshed. However, a little sport can let you feel the morning freshness. You will be more relaxed and have more energy for the day.

On the following pages, I will introduce you to a well thought out and balanced early morning sport programme, that will make you fit for the day.

A 10 MINUTE MORNING EXERCISE

This exercise is guaranteed to boost your energy levels. It consists of 10 single exercises, which only take one minute each. They become increasingly difficult. It is suitable for the morning exercise unit or as a warm-up for more strenuous training units.

I carried out my morning sport unit with this exercise as a starting point. Because it is short and intensive, it was exactly the right thing for me. After that, I significantly increased my morning training. Now I use this exercise as my warm-up before I do my longer sport programme.

Watch out! If you have been neglecting your sporting activity lately, it is quite possible, that you will experience muscle stiffness the next morning. The more often you do sport, the less muscle stiffness you will experience.

1. *Grabbing while on your toes*
   Stretching in the morning is ideal for waking up your spirits.

For this exercise, you will stretch alternately one arm upwards then the other, while bringing down the opposite arm, slightly bent, to your side. You will experience a pleasant stretching feeling in your body.

Go up onto your toes every time you stretch an arm upwards.

2. *Circling shoulders backwards*

This exercise loosens your shoulder joints and is very good for avoiding shoulder tension, particularly if you work at a desk.

For this exercise, you rotate your hands outwards as far as you can, and then make circles of the shoulder joints, backwards.

Everyday tip: This exercise is suitable to do, when you need it, in a seated position, perhaps at your desk, in order to loosen your shoulders.

3. *Stretching arms around you*

For this exercise you will draw as big a circle as possible in the air, around your body.

Stretch one arm in front of your body and turn your palm upwards.

With your arm straight, draw the biggest circle you can, upwards at an angle of 45° behind your head and back down the other side while your body remains facing forwards. Keep your palms facing upwards. At the end of the circle, bend your arm towards you and under the armpit in order to close the circle. After about half a minute, change arms and do the same thing with the other arm.

4. *Arched back and hollow back*

For this exercise you bend your knees slightly and push your spine upwards, arching your back. Lower your back to sink into the hollow position.

Allow your head to go with the movement as well as your hips. While the back is arched, lower your head, looking towards your feet. While the back is hollow, look upwards.

As an alternative, you can do this exercise on all fours.

5. *Eagle's wings*

For this exercise you should stand with your feet wide apart and make squats.

Stretch your arms out to the sides like an eagle when you do your next knee-bend. When you come back up, sink your arms once more.

Ensure your back is straight and lower your buttocks as much as your strength and mobility will allow.

6. *Lunges with rotation*

Make a lunge, that means make a large step forwards with the right foot and your body, simultaneously.

Turn to the left side, so that you rotate your upper body. Stretch both your arms out, parallel to your legs.

Stand back up and repeat the exercise. Start this time with the left foot. Carry out this exercise alternatively with the right and left foot.

The rotating movement will ensure good flexibility to your spine.

7. *Crab Reach*

Sit with your buttocks on the floor, then press your hips upwards with your hands and feet. Resting on one arm, stretch the other arm backwards, behind your head.

Come back to the position on the floor, then press your hips once again, this time stretching your other arm backwards.

This exercise helps to alleviate the problems caused by sitting all day.

8. *Wild cat push up*

From here onwards, you will notice, that the exercises become more difficult.

Start in the "push up" position. Move backwards to sit on your heels, making sure not to touch the floor with your knees.

Move back down into the "push up" position and do one push up. Repeat the exercise for a minute.

This way, you improve your body tone and train your arm and chest muscles.

9. *The Cassowary kick*

Get into a straddle position, put your hands on the ground. Push a leg through the gap between your arms and other leg and lower your buttocks to the ground.

During this exercise, only the hands and one foot are on the ground. The other, stretched foot stays above the ground.

This exercise is perfect for giving your stomach muscles that burning feeling.

10. *The awakening dog*

Slowly, we are getting to the end of the exercises. Let us now do the awaking and sniffing dog, so that we are wide awake.

Go to the starting position: Hands and feet on the ground, facing downwards, pushing the buttocks up as far as possible.

Sink your face towards the ground and, without touching the ground, lead the body weight forwards and upwards into an arched position.

Come back the same way, leading with the nose along the ground like a sniffing dog while you come back to the start position.

RELAXATION TECHNIQUES

In addition to sport in the morning, other activities, which can bring your body and mind in harmony, can be very useful. Exercises you can include range from autogenic training, Jacobson's progressive muscle relaxation or breathing exercises to meditation or yoga. It could be a combination of two or more of these.

Also, after you have finished with your fitness training, relaxation is very important for the body and mind. The relaxation techniques, such as meditation and yoga can be learned quickly, without specific training. However, it is of course an advantage, if you can learn from a professional. That way, you receive specific tips and improvement suggestions.

There are some suitable techniques on the following pages.

THE SUN SALUTATION

The yoga sun salutation is suitable to carry out after getting up in order to waken your spirit or as a warm up for a yoga stint or a sport unit.

According to yoga practice, the sequence of the positions in the sun salutation, otherwise known as Surya Namaskar, follows the flow of your own breath.

Carrying out this exercise is invigorating for the body, soul and spirit. You mobilise your joints, stretch your muscles and ligaments and train your cardiovascular system. There are many variations of the sun salutation.

I will explain the sequence of Sun Salutation A, for beginners. I do this exercise several times each day after getting up. It is up to you how many times you repeat the exercise. In the internet, there are many videos about it, which can help you at the start, so that you can see how to complete the exercise correctly.

1. <u>The mountain pose</u>
    - To begin, bring yourself to the front edge of the yoga mat.

- Stand, legs hip-width apart, the insides of the feet are parallel to each other.
- Imagine a thread, which is pulling the back of your head slightly upwards.
- Tip your pelvis slightly forwards to prevent hollowing your back.
- Let your arms rest, relaxed, beside your body, the palms facing forwards.

2. *Extended mountain pose*
   - Take a deep breath.
   - Bring your arms out to the sides and upwards, so that the palms touch.
   - Look up at your hands.
   - Keep your abdomen firm and allow your tailbone to sink slightly.
   - Relax your neck and shoulders and let them sink back down again.

3. *Whole forward bend*
   - Breathe out.

- Bend the whole upper body from the hips forwards and downwards.
- Touch the floor with your hands.
- If possible, keep your legs stretched, if not the knees can remain a little bent.
- Relax your upper body, lengthen your neck.

4. *Half forward bend*
   - Take a deep breath.
   - Lift your upper body so that it makes a 90° angle.
   - Point the arms and fingers downwards without touching the ground.
   - Concentrate on the length of your upper body.

5. *Upward plank*
   - Breathe out.
   - Lower your hands to the mat.
   - Put one leg, then the other, into the push up position.

- Spread your fingers and ensure they are under your shoulders. Pull your shoulders together, keep your abdomen firm.
- The toes are on the ground, heels in the air.
- Maintain a straight line with your back.
- Breathe in and hold your breath.

6. *Face down*
   - Breathe out.
   - Lower your knees to the ground.
   - Allow your body to return, controlled, to the mat.
   - Rest your forehead on the mat, draw your elbows tightly towards your body. Draw your naval to your backbone.

7. *Small Cobra*
   - Breathe in deeply.
   - Lift your upper body.

- Let your neck sink slowly and look upwards.
- Press your pubic bone and toes into the mat.
- Draw your elbows close to your body.

8. *Face down*
   - Breathe out.
   - Let your body return, controlled, onto the mat.
   - Concentrate on the length of your body.
   - Rest your forehead on the mat. Draw your elbows close to your body, and the naval to the backbone.

9. *Downward-facing dog*
   - Breathe in deeply.
   - As you are breathing, bend your toes and push your buttocks towards your heels.
   - Your forehead is facing downwards.

- Breathe out
- Slowly stretch your legs and arrive in the position of the downward-facing dog.
- Divide your weight evenly between your arms and legs.
- Face downwards.
- Breath in deeply.

10. *Whole forward bend*
    - Breathe out.
    - While breathing out, take a big step to the forward edge of the mat.
    - Bend your whole body from the hips forwards and downwards.
    - Touch the floor with your hands.
    - Let your head hang downwards.

11. *Half forward bend*
    - Breath in deeply.
    - As you are breathing in, bend your body, so that it makes a 90° angle.

- Your arms and fingers should be pointing towards the ground but not touching it.
- Concentrate on the length of your upper body.

12. <u>Whole forward bend</u>
    - Breathe out.
    - While breathing out, bend your whole body from the hips forwards and downwards.
    - Touch the floor with your hands.
    - Relax your upper body, stretch your neck.

13. <u>Extended mountain pose</u>
    - Breathe in deeply.
    - Bring your arms out to the sides and upwards so that the palms touch.
    - Look up at your hands
    - Keep your abdomen firm and allow your tailbone to sink slightly.

- Relax your neck and shoulders and let them sink back down again.

14. *The mountain pose*
    - Breathe out.
    - While breathing out, lower your arms to your sides.
    - Place your palms together in front of your chest in a prayer-like posture.
    - Look forwards.

FIVE MOTIVATION TIPS

In the following pages, I will give you five important tips, which will help you to motivate yourself, to put into practice your newly-learned daily routine and how not to fall back into your old behavioural routines.

Of course, there are many other ideas, which you can discover, in order to make yourself a long-term early bird.

USE THE QUIET TIME

It is a great advantage to be first up in the morning: You are alone. That means, you can concentrate on what you are doing and remain focused on yourself. There are no mobile phones, fellow occupants or neighbours, who can distract or interrupt you.

Would you prefer to do some jogging? Then you would not want to swap the peace of a morning jog for anything. The atmosphere in the morning is indescribable. The streets are still quiet and the pavements are void of people. You and the open road. A relaxation technique or meditation in the park while it is still quiet and with chirping birds and other natural sounds is also very beneficial and helps you to relax more fully.

In the early morning, you are the only one about. You with your clear thoughts, your aims and your plans. Use this time for yourself.

BOOST YOUR METABOLISM

You activate your metabolism in the morning as soon as you start moving. If you boost it with a sport programme in the morning, followed by a wholesome breakfast, it will continue to work hard for you the whole day. The better your metabolism works, the better you are able to process your nutrition and provide energy for your body during the day.

DISCIPLINE

Do you recognise the following excuses you make before doing your evening sport? Too tired from work, a meeting with friends, unfinished jobs, things you need to attend to, doing the washing, shopping etc.? In the evening, the chances are much higher of you concentrating on other things, rather than sport.

Do you feel drained in the evenings? Not enough concentration for a meditation? Then try it in the mornings, while you are still fresh. Once you are awake, it is easier to reach for your training shoes and yoga mat, because all the things you did not have time to do in the evenings are no problem in the morning. Your mind is still free and receptive. Your self-discipline is at its strongest in the morning. This should enable you to be more successful in your efforts.

Once you have shown the discipline to carry out what you intended to do, a few days in a row, you can see, that it becomes easier as time goes on. Keep at it!

BE SUCCESSFUL

If you start your day the way you intended, you can already celebrate your first success. You radiate serenity and tranquillity and this projects in a very positive way onto other people. Your mind is clearer, your body is fitter and this leads to success in everyday life. This success has a knock-on effect and will continue to grow: But be careful, this also works the other way around, so stay true to your aims and do not allow yourself any slack with your new routines.

FEELING HAPPY ALL DAY

Use the morning, and the time you have before the day really begins, to do the things, which make you feel better, which motivate you and which give you inspiration and energy. The fact, that the others are still lying in bed and are wasting this valuable part of the day, while you are active, gives you a good feeling and motivates you, does not it?

No one can take that feeling of happiness away from you. You take it with you to work and it accompanies you throughout the day.

Perhaps you feel like me and never want to do without it again in the future. You get up full of motivation and fully intend to get the best out of your day.

- Chapter 7 -

THE EARLY BIRD CHALLENGE IN 10 STEPS

Are you thinking, that even after reading all this information, you still have not heard specifically how you can become an early bird? Everything you have read up to now is very important for you. Knowledge is the first step towards change, the basis upon which we form an understanding about what happens to us and how we react. Now you can use everything you have learned to become an early bird.

The background knowledge, that I gained about the sleep-wake rhythm, for example, has led me to re-think everything. I plan my sleeping times completely different and I use the knowledge I have gained to avoid being woken up sharply from the deepest of sleeps.

Now it is your turn to change your habits and to become an early bird. Undertake to wake up early and at the same time every day over the next 30 days. I am convinced, that after 30 days you will want to continue with your new habit when you have experienced the advantages.

The exact time you should wake up, is up to you, but I recommend waking up at least 1 to 2 hours before you normally do, so that you have enough time to try out your new routine and leave the house fit and awake.

In the following pages, I will introduce you to 10 important steps explaining how you can become an early bird:

STEP 1: FIND A REASON TO GET UP IN THE MORNING

Who gets up in the morning without a reason? No one. You need motivation and purpose to get out of bed. What do you want to achieve at work today?

Formulate a purpose for you personally. What is your incentive/motivation for becoming an early bird? Your aims should encompass the following points (for example according to the SMART rules)

- *Specific:*
  Formulate specific objectives that you want to achieve. Avoid generalities, it is better to set several aims rather than one primary goal.

- *Measurable:*
  Specify timings. Cross-check real times with projected ones.

- *Attractive/Acceptable:*
  Choose a goal, which makes sense for you and which is acceptable to others. Early morning

Zumba training, for example, would not go down well with other occupants or neighbours.

- *Realistic:*
  Your goal should be realistic. It is better to make smaller, achievable goals rather than one which you are not sure you can achieve.

- *Timed:*
  Use deadlines, such as a period of time by which you want to achieve your goal. This gives you a point of comparison between your achievement and your goal.

To help you picture it better, here is an example of one of the goals that I started with: "I will get up at 7am every working day for the next 30 days and do yoga exercises for 30 minutes."

Avoid negatives at all costs when setting out your goals. Our brain has the habit of switching off or erasing "do not" or "none". The content that we want to avoid is all that our subconscious recognises in the sentence. In addition, the negation reminds you of forbidding something and is not particularly motivating. "I do not want to stay in bed any more until 9am" could, for example, be changed into the following sentence: "I will get up every day at 7am."

STEP 2: FIND YOUR NEW SLEEPING RHYTHM

I am sure you know the feeling when you are deeply asleep and the alarm goes off. At first, you are completely disoriented and not sure where you are, let alone what is happening. It is very difficult for you to open your eyelids and to wake up. This is due to your sleep phases or rather your sleep cycle. You have probably been ripped out of a deep-sleep phase. Your sleeping cycle was not completed and it is particularly difficult to get up during that phase.

SLEEP LESS THROUGH CORRECT SLEEP

There is a trick to help you achieve your goal: Less sleep through correct sleep! Understanding the sleep phases and cycles, you will be able to get up better, even if you get less sleep. If you wake up at the right time, that means at the end of the 6th sleeping phase, instead of in the deep-sleep phase, you will have more energy and not feel as if you have been run over by a steamroller. All you need to do is to adapt your sleeping times to your sleeping phases.

In the next section, you will find an example table divided into hourly segments. The table also works in half-hour or quarter-hour segments. In order to save space, I have kept to the full hours. All you need to do is reduce it by the time it takes to go to sleep, for example, by 15 minutes.

Sleep begin:	9pm	10pm	11pm	12pm
1st Cycle	10:30	11:30	00:30	01:30
2nd Cycle	00:00	01:30	02:30	03:30

3rd Cycle	01:30	02:30	03:30	04:30
4th Cycle	03:00	04:00	05:00	06:00
5th Cycle	04:30	05:30	06:30	07:30
6th Cycle	06:00	07:00	08:00	09:00

Say, for example, you want to wake up at 7am and you need about 15 minutes to go to sleep. This means for you that your ideal 'sleep begin' time would be 10 pm, minus the 15 minutes that you need to go to sleep – that would mean 9.45pm. Should you miss your sleeping time, the next opportunity would be 11.30pm, minus 15 minutes that you need to go to sleep – which would mean 11.15pm.

This seems to be complicated at first, but really it is quite simple. You just have to divide your sleeping time by 1.5 hours (90 minutes). A healthy sleep length could therefore be either 6 hours, 7.5 hours or 9 hours etc. In the internet there are sleep calculators, which can help you calculate it at the beginning.

Naturally, every sleep cycle can have its anomalies, so you just need to try it out. Keep a note of your sleep begin time and your waking up time at the beginning, together with a comment about how you feel. This way, it is easier to find out your ideal bedtime. Sometimes only a small difference can make a big impact as to whether you feel top fit at the end of a sleeping cycle or are dead tired and in the middle of a deep sleep phase.

STEP 3: ESTABLISH YOUR MORNING ROUTINE

You can determine how your morning routine will look. You will only be successful, if you plan it yourself. Despite that, you can be inspired by successful early birds, who can help to show you what a morning routine could look like.

In the next chapter I will introduce you to a strategy from Hal Elrod. This is the person, who inspired my personal morning routine.

S.A.V.E.R. BY ELROD

The American bestseller author, Hal Elrod presented his strategy for a morning routine in his bestseller book: "Miracle Morning. The 6 habits that will transform your life before 8am". A strategy which he developed for his morning routine, which lasts 90 minutes.

Elrod recommends 6 habits for the morning that he calls "life-S.A.V.E.R.S". It involves a mixture between relaxation and activity.

S = Silence – 5 minutes:
Use the quiet first peaceful 5 minutes for breathing exercises or meditation.

A = Affirmations – 5 minutes:
Use affirmations to influence your subconscious mind.

Affirmations are positive tenets, which can be carried out in in different ways. For example, you can say them out loud, write them down or play them from a pre-recorded sound file. It is a kind of positive persuasion, a confirmation in words of your objective. For it to work, it is important, that the affirmation is convincing and that it comes from you.

V = Visualisation – 10 minutes
Stay aware of your objectives, create pictures in your head or with the help of drawings.

Visualising is about using your own imagination effectively, in order to portray your thoughts, ideas and messaging. Doing this makes the invisible become visible, objectives become clearer and take a more specific form. The incomprehensible becomes palpable and you can give the vagueness a sharper contour.

E = Exercise (sport)– 30 minutes
Reserve a half-hour for sporting activity, such as jogging, yoga, or body workout. You can decide for yourself which you choose.

Reading – 30 minutes
Read something inspiring in the morning.

S = Scribing – 10 minutes
Put your thoughts, ideas and targets on paper. It could be a kind of diary where you write everything down,

that is on your mind and what you aspire to i.e. what you want to achieve.

STEP 4: DEFINE YOUR EVENING ROUTINE

"A good day begins the evening before". This means, that your morning routine and the coming day can only be successful with the right evening programme.

Getting up earlier means going to bed earlier, whether we like it or not. If you are an owl, it will probably be quite difficult for you to go to bed early and settle down at the beginning.

Perhaps you are also thinking, that you will have to reduce your social activities because you cannot stay up late with your friends. If you can bring your activities forwards a little, there is no reason why you cannot meet your friends. As you have done your yoga or fitness session early in the morning, you will have more time in the evening to do other things.

TIPS TO CALM DOWN IN THE EVENING

You have already planned your morning routine, and taking your sleep phases and sleep cycles into consideration, you have set an ideal time for you to go to bed. Do not push this back to a later time. Start your evening routine early enough so that you do not miss your bed time.

Here are a few ideas, which may help you to come to rest.

Relaxation:
A relaxing yoga, meditation or relaxation technique may help you to calm down. Also playing relaxing music in the background, while you are carrying out an activity or reading, may also help. Everyone has their own preferences, find out what helps you to switch off.

You can also carry out relaxation techniques, such as autogenic training or Jacobson's progressive muscle relaxation in bed, before you go to sleep. There are instruction programmes, which you can play on an MP3 player. Listening to the voice of the instructor can help you, if you are not yet well-practised in these techniques.

Dimmed lights:
As you already know, we need the darkness so that our bodies begin with the production of the sleeping hormone, Melatonin. Make sure you dim the lights in the living room and avoid working on your laptop late at night.

I always switch on the blue light filter of my smartphone in the afternoons. My laptop and E-reader also have this feature, although not every device does. If you have it, use it, to decrease the blue light as much as possible.

Say goodbye to the digital world:
Define a time of day when you always turn your smartphone onto flight mode, or set yourself a reminder. Social media, surfing the internet, checking emails and looking at news can all feel relaxing but information is constantly filling your brain and making it more difficult to go to sleep. Also, vibration and signal tones can disturb your relaxation, shortly before sleeping and can cause you to reach for your smartphone.

My family and friends have got used to the idea, that my smartphone is on flight mode from 9pm onwards and I am no longer available, so they are not surprised, if they do not receive an answer.

Drinking before sleep:
Warm milk with honey or an infusion with a calming effect can help you to go off to sleep. Do not drink directly before going to bed. Give it time to do its work before turning in. This way, you can also avoid having to get up to use the bathroom in the night, which may disturb your rest. Naturally, it all depends on the amount. Drinking too much within a short time is also not particularly conducive to good sleep.

Reading / Listening to audio books:
Instead of spending your evening in front of a monitor, reading or listening to audio books can be a good alternative. Make sure you have a good reading light, which ensures enough light to read with but does not fill the room with bright light. E-readers with the nightlight mode option are a good alternative. Audio books are also a good alternative, because they give out no light and you can go to sleep in the dark while listening to your story on your MP3 player.

Walking in the evening:
Taking a walk at dusk can help your body produce the Melatonin you need for sleep in a natural way. In addition, light exercise and fresh air can help to free your mind. Allow your thoughts to fly away with every step.

Reflect on the day:
Every day we are subject to many stimuli and impressions. Allowing yourself to relive the day in the evenings can help you to find your peace. You can either do that with your partner, or other occupant, or by writing into a diary.

Affirmations:
Repeat your positive affirmations before you go to sleep. Listening to them, reading them through or writing them down helps you to internalise them and let them sink into your subconscious. I do this when I am already in bed and I look forward to the positive things in my life.

STEP 5: PREPARATION IS EVERYTHING

Getting up early also means using the time properly. I recommend making preparations the night before, so that you do not waste any time in the morning. For example, you can lay out your clothes or sport equipment, ready for the next day.

You can also make preparations for your breakfast. For example, you can prepare your oats or chia pudding for your muesli to steep overnight.

I always roll out my yoga mat and put out my clothes the previous evening, so that I do not dawdle in doing that in the morning.

STEP 6: OPTIMISE YOUR ALARM SYSTEM

Some people swear by their light alarms. If you do not already possess one, you can perhaps change your waking tone or place your alarm clock in a more optimal position. As I already mentioned, vigorous songs are best. Choose one that motivates you to begin your day.

If you are chronic "snoozer", place your alarm out of arm's reach, so that you are forced to get up.

STEP 7: GET STRAIGHT OUT OF BED

Get out of bed straight away when your alarm rings. Do not be tempted to lie down again. Daylight helps to wake you up, open the curtains, even if it is still dark at that moment, and open the window for a portion of fresh air. Fill your lungs with fresh oxygen and awaken your spirits.

Perhaps it helps to jump straight into the shower to wake up better. I prefer to go straight into the bathroom and wash my face with cold water. Then I shower after I have done my sport. That way, my eyes do not feel so swollen and heavy. Once you are on your feet and have started your routine, you will no longer be thinking of going back to bed.

STEP 8: PLAN YOUR WEEKENDS MEANINGFULLY

Maintain your new sleeping rhythm unequivocally for the next 30 days, also at the weekends. You will need continuity, so that your body can get used to the new rhythm.

Is your motivation less than favourable for getting up early at the weekends? This should not be the case, because your new rhythm has so many advantages. You can get so much more out of your days. If you get up at 6am and go to work at 8am during the week, you have the time from 8am at the weekends to do the things you usually leave until the afternoon. You will probably be finished with all of those things by the afternoon and then have the rest of the day to do something you want to do. Meet your friends in the mornings or afternoons, if possible, so that you can go to bed early. That way, you are not losing the time you have for social contacts. You just need to organise them differently.

STEP 9: KEEP AT IT!

Today, you are probably full of motivation to change something in your life. The challenge is yet to come: That is to keep at it. Many people give up after a few days and go back to their old routines. The following 6 points will help you to avoid that and to be more successful at staying an early bird:

1. *Start right now:*

Use the next 72 hours to put into practice, what you have learned. Studies have shown, that 99% of all intensions and aims, which are not started within the first 72 hours, are never implemented. So best begin immediately!

2. *No exceptions:*

If you make an exception once, you run the danger of being tempted again. Do not even start with that and be proud, that you reach your target every day.

3. *More motivation with a partner:*

Find a partner with whom you can do a quick round of jogging with, because this is an ideal motivation.

Once you have made the arrangements to meet, you cannot get out of it very easily.

4. *Share experiences:*

Sharing your experiences and success with others can be immensely motivating and stimulating. Tell your friends and colleagues about your morning routine and what you have been able to improve with it. There may even be someone who will follow your example.

5. *Don't overdo it:*

Do not overreach yourself. Do not plan too many things into your morning routine, start slowly. Planning too many things can impede your motivation, because it makes your morning too stressful. Start slowly and add other habits to it over time.

6. *Do not be disheartened*

Did you not manage to keep to your morning routine? Do not give up on your intentions straight away. It is clearly difficult to give up your old habits and substitute them with new ones. Do not let setbacks dishearten you. Stay motivated and try again the next morning.

STEP 10: ENJOY YOUR NEW LIFE AS AN EARLY BIRD

That is the most important point of all. Be proud of yourself. You have managed to change your old habits successfully. The extra hours, that you have won, can be the most productive of the whole day and will eventually be something you will not want to do without. Now you are conscious of all the hours you used to waste. No one can take away all the advantages you have as an early bird. Enjoy every day and begin each day full of zest.

- Chapter 8 -

CONCLUSION

Knowing about the sleep phases and cycles was one of the most important factors, which helped me to succeed. Adjusting my sleeping time to my physical rhythm enabled me to get up much more easily in the mornings. It sounds simple to find out when the most ideal sleeping time for you should be, using a calculator. In fact, it takes some time to find out what is ideal for you, personally. Getting up to go to the bathroom in the middle of the night and taking a long time to go back to sleep could change your sleeping cycle, as an example. Despite that, it can be useful in planning your sleeping times. If you miss your time for going to bed, I recommend waiting until the end of that cycle and going to bed 1.5 hours later. Then you are sure to get up in the morning at the end of a sleeping cycle.

The "Life-S.A.V.E.R.S" strategy from Hal Elrod inspired me to plan my morning routine and make the most of the extra time. Personally, I felt that so many changes from one routine to another were too much in the morning. I altered the concept to suit my own needs. I like to finish my sporting activity with a meditation. Meditating directly upon waking up did not suit me, because I was still too sleepy and the temptation to go back to bed was too great. After the meditation, I go in the shower and repeat my affirmations.

As I already mentioned, I love to read. Therefore, I often combine this activity with my breakfast. If I still have time, I spend it on writing my diary or in visualising my goals more tangibly by representing my thoughts with abstract drawings in my dairy. My morning routine takes about 90 minutes, as does Elrod's strategy, but this includes the shower and breakfast.

After I had finished my early bird challenge, and got used to my new daily routine, I was even able to put my getting up time an hour earlier. So, now I go to bed at about 10.15pm and get up at 6am. My morning routine takes 90 minutes, so that I am top fit at 7.30am to begin my work. In comparison, I used to get up at 9am and still needed a few minutes before I could start my work. These days, I am much more productive, more concentrated and more efficient in my work. I am not the only one, who has noticed this. My employer and my team colleagues have also noticed positive changes.

It does not matter whether you are more sporting in the morning or prefer to do more relaxing activities, the peaceful morning atmosphere is priceless and no one can take it away from us. What other time of day can we concentrate on only ourselves, undisturbed and in peace, whether it be a sport programme, yoga or meditation? I am able to draw on more energy at this time than any other time of the day. The external noise is low and there are hardly any interruptions, which can cause a distraction.

I have succeeded in changing from a late-riser to an early bird. The most important factor was how I went about my early bird challenge. I failed on my first attempt, because I did not have a proper plan and not enough knowledge about my physical rhythms. However, I am sure, with the right preparation, willpower and motivation, anyone can become an early bird. With this book and through other means, I am trying to reach as many people as I can to tell them, that it is possible.

I hope your early bird challenge ends positively and you are able to make the necessary changes to lead a more successful and happy life. I wish you luck!

DID YOU ENJOY MY BOOK?

Now you have read my book you know how to become an early bird in no time and how to use your morning routine to lead to a more fulfilling life. This is why I am asking you now for a small favour. Customer reviews are an important part of every product offered by Amazon. It is the first thing that customers look at and, more often than not, is the main reason whether or not they decide to buy the product. Considering the endless number of products available at Amazon, this factor is becoming increasingly important.

If you liked my book, I would be more than grateful if you could leave your review by Amazon. How do you do that? Just click on the "Write a customer review"-button (as shown below), which you find on the Amazon product page of my book or your orders site:

Review this product

Share your thoughts with other customers

Write a customer review

Please write a short note explaining what you liked most and what you found to be most important. It will not take longer than a few minutes, promise!

Be assured, I will read every review personally. It will help me a lot to improve my books and to tailor them to your wishes.

For this I say to you:

Thank you very much!

Yours
Lutz

BOOK RECOMMENDATIONS

LUTZ SCHNEIDER

THE POWER OF BREATHING TECHNIQUES

Breathing Exercises for more Fitness, Health and Relaxation

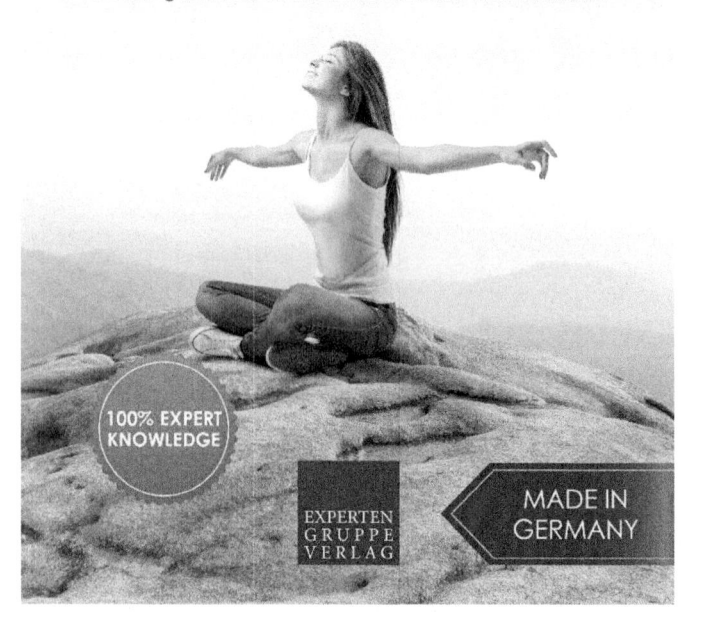

100% EXPERT KNOWLEDGE

EXPERTEN GRUPPE VERLAG

MADE IN GERMANY

The Power of Breathing Techniques

Breathing Exercises for more Fitness, Health and Relaxation

We can survive for weeks without food and days without water, but only a few minutes without air.

Would it not be justified to presume that the air, which is more important for human survival than food or water, should live up to basic standards? How much air do we need for ideal breathing? And how should we breathe?

The amount of air that you breathe has the potential to change everything you believe about your body, your health and your performance.

In this book, you will discover the fundamental relationship between Oxygen and your body.

Increasing your Oxygen supply is not only healthy, it enables an increase in the intensity of your training and also reduces breathlessness. In short, you will notice an improvement in your health and more relaxation in your everyday life.

Look forward to reading a lot of background information, experience reports, step-by-step instructions and secret tips which are tailor-made to your breathing technique and help you to become fitter, healthier and more relaxed.

This book is available on Amazon!

LUTZ SCHNEIDER

LITHIUM
AND
LITHIUM CARBONATE

A MEDICINAL PRODUCT FOR DEPRESSION, ALZHEIMER AND DEMENTIA, FOR IMPROVING WELL-BEING AND MANAGING STRESS

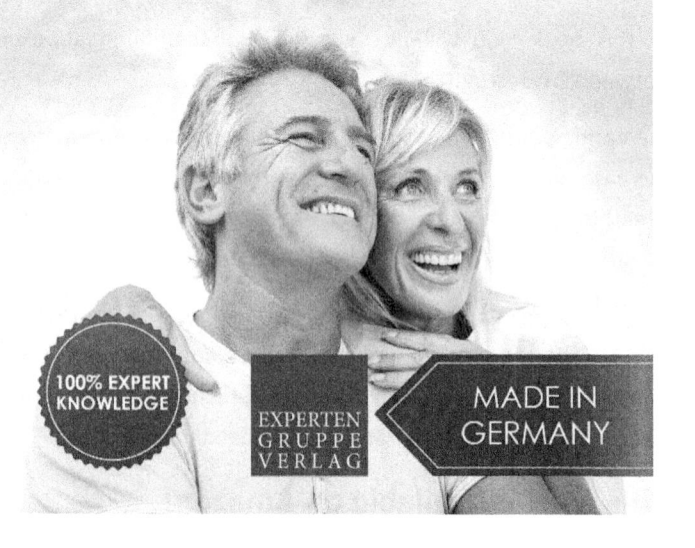

100% EXPERT KNOWLEDGE

EXPERTEN GRUPPE VERLAG

MADE IN GERMANY

Lithium and Lithium Carbonate

A medicinal product for Depression, Alzheimer and Dementia, for improving well-being and managing stress

Lithium is mostly known for its use in batteries. Most people do not realise that it is also a trace element in our bodies.

Would it not be wonderful if you could fight sicknesses, such as depression or Alzheimer, and improve your well-being, if you just had a little more Lithium in your body? What if you did not have to do anything more than take a little more Lithium?

Lithium is an important component for all of us in achieving a lasting, healthy way of life. Clinical studies and scientific articles are speaking a clear language. Despite that, Lithium is suffering a niche existence by a large majority of pharmaceutical scientists and is hardly known by the broad population.

Even so, the advantages of Lithium, which lie in psychological and mental health sector, are obvious and it is easy to obtain and use.

In this book, you will discover the advantages and effects of Lithium on your body and mind.

Read about fascinating background information, scientific findings, experience reports and secret tips which are tailor-made for your needs and which will help you to achieve a healthy, longer and more fulfilling life.

This book is available on Amazon!

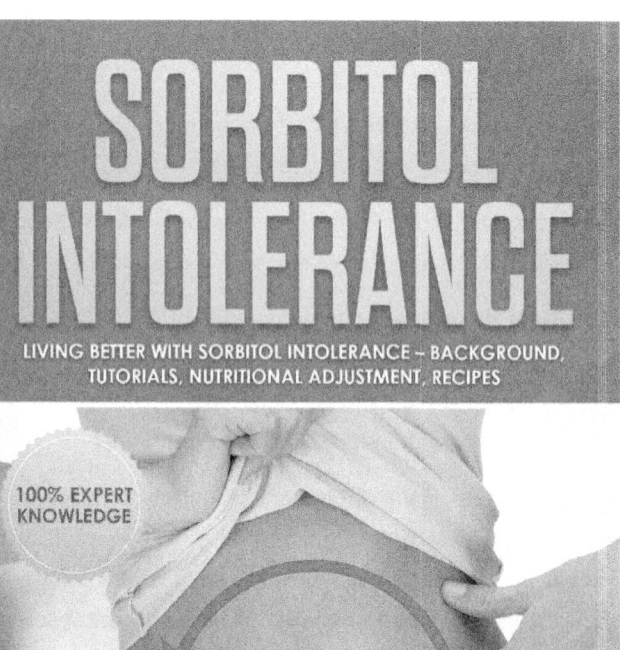

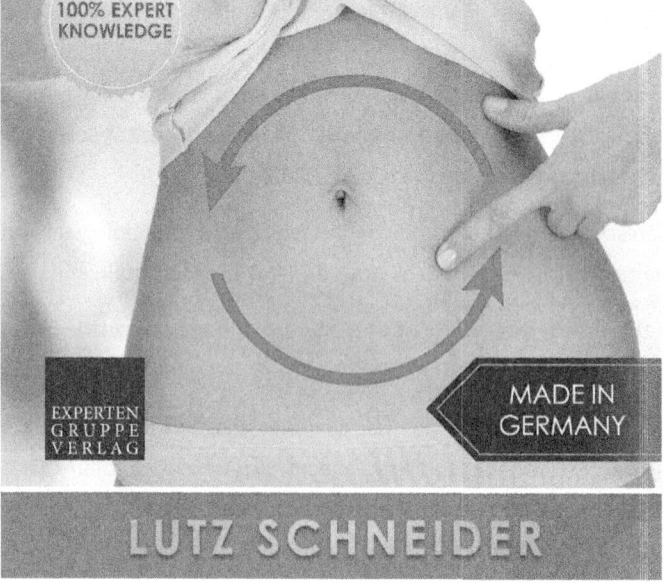

SORBITOL INTOLERANCE

LIVING BETTER WITH SORBITOL INTOLERANCE – BACKGROUND, TUTORIALS, NUTRITIONAL ADJUSTMENT, RECIPES

100% EXPERT KNOWLEDGE

EXPERTEN GRUPPE VERLAG

MADE IN GERMANY

LUTZ SCHNEIDER

Sorbitol Intolerance

Living better with Sorbitol intolerance – background, tutorials, nutritional adjustment, recipes

Sorbitol intolerance is one of the least known food intolerances among many. And that, even though more and more people are suffering from it.

Wouldn't it be wonderful if you could at last find out if you suffer from Sorbitol intolerance? And how can you eat a diverse and delicious diet, despite your Sorbitol intolerance?

An increasing amount of industrially prepared food means that more and more people are taking doses of Sorbitol which they are not able to digest properly. This leads to a large number of lingering symptoms which are difficult to assign to any particular substance.

In this book you will find a simple guide on how to change your diet and a lot of important information about the subject of Sorbitol.

Read about fascinating background information, scientific findings, experience reports and secret tips which are tailor-made for you relating to your Sorbitol intolerance and which are designed to help you to achieve a healthy, longer and more fulfilling life.

This book is available on Amazon!

LIST OF REFERENCES

Besser schlafen: sanfte Wege zu einer erholsamen Nacht,
1. Aufl. von Pütz, Jean Fricke, Sabine Pohl, Monika, 2000

Endlich wieder gut schlafen: Schlafen lernen, Schlafstörungen beseitigen
von Schneider, Ute, 2001

Wieder gut schlafen können: was Sie gegen Ein- und Durchschlafprobleme tun können
von Feld, Karsten, 1994

Endlich wieder schlafen können: ohne Medikamente gut schlafen; das erfolgreiche Selbsthilfe-Programm
von Coates, Thomas J Thoresen, Carl E, 1982

Endlich erholsam schlafen
von Chopra, Deepak
1994

Schlaf: Gehirnaktivität im Ruhezustand
von Hobson, J. Allan, 1990

Untersuchung zum Schlafverhalten von Schülern der Gymnasialen Oberstufe an einem beispielhaften Versuchsobjekt: Von Eulen und Lerchen
1. Aufl., von Blefgen, Carolin, 2011

Schlafgewohnheiten und Schlafqualität: Von der späten Kindheit bis ins Erwachsenenalter
1. Aufl., von Strauch, Inge, 2010

JuSt - Therapeutenmanual : Das Training für Jugendliche ab 11 Jahren mit Schlafstörungen
von Schlarb, Angelika, 2015

Karrierefaktor Guter Schlaf : Wie Sie Sich Zu Höchstleistungen Schlummern
von Pohl, Elke, 2015

Schluss mit Schlafproblemen : So verbessern Sie Ihre Schlafqualität und Ihr Wohlbefinden
von Jahn, Ruth Mathis, Johannes Roth, Corinne, 2014

Warum Schlafmangel dick und guter Schlaf schlank macht
von Worm, Nicolai, 2016

https://flexikon.doccheck.com/de/Zirkadianer_Rhythmus

https://www.stern.de/gesundheit/schlaf/geheimnis_schlaf/schlafrhythmus-wie-unsere-innere-uhr-tickt-3762946.htmlSchlafphasen

https://www.zeit.de/zeit-wissen/2008/02/Zeit

https://www.habitgym.de/fruehaufsteher-werden/

https://www.rnz.de/zeitjung_artikel,-beginn-des-schulunterrichts-die-eulen-haben-durchgehend-schlechtere-noten-_arid,301312.html

https://www.helsana.ch/de/blog/welcher-schlaftyp-sind-sie

https://www.derschlafraum.de/blog/die-fuenf-schlafphasen-so-sieht-gesunder-schlaf-aus/

https://utopia.de/ratgeber/besser-schlafen-tipp-abendroutine-schlafhygiene/

https://www.spektrum.de/news/was-bei-schlafmangel-im-gehirn-passiert/1560834

https://www.4yourfitness.com/blog/fruehsport-uebungen

https://www.gesundheit.de/krankheiten/gehirn-und-nerven/schlafstoerungen/schlaf-warum-schlafen-wir

https://www.netdoktor.de/schlaf/schlaftypen-von-eulen-und-ler-11355.html

https://www.sueddeutsche.de/gesundheit/schlafforschung-wie-viel-schlaf-ist-optimal-1.4164426

https://www.motivate-yourself.de/schlafzyklen-nutzen-schlaf-optimieren/

https://www.t-online.de/gesundheit/krankheiten-symptome/id_81354606/was-zu-wenig-schlaf-mit-unserem-koerper-macht.html

https://www.der-bank-blog.de/fruehaufsteher-langschlaefer/fuehrung-und-management/37107/

https://karrierebibel.de/morgenroutine/#Erklaerung-Was-ist-eine-Morgenroutine-ueberhaupt

https://arbeits-abc.de/morgenroutine-fuer-mehr-erfolg/

https://utopia.de/ratgeber/koffein-wirkung-nebenwirkung-und-was-du-sonst-noch-wissen-solltest/

https://www.meine-gesundheit.de/ratgeber/schlaf/schlaf-essen-trinken

https://www.evidero.de/sport-am-morgen

https://www.stern.de/gesundheit/miracle-morning--jeden-tag-eine-stunde-frueher-aufstehen--um-wacher-zu-sein-7922474.html

DISCLAIMER

©2020, Lutz Schneider

1st Edition

All rights reserved. Reprinting, of all or part of this book, is not permitted. No part of this book may be reproduced or copied in any form or by any means without written permission from the author or publisher. Publisher: GbR, Martin Seidel und Corinna Krupp, Bachstraße 37, 53498 Bad Breisig, Germany, email: info@expertengruppeverlag.de, Cover photo: www.depositphoto.com. The information provided within this book is for general information purposes only. It does not represent any recommendation or application of the methods mentioned within. The information in this book does not purport to imply or guarantee its completeness, accuracy, or topicality. This book in no way replaces the competent recommendations of, or care given by, a doctor. The author and publisher do not assume and hereby disclaims any liability for damages or disruption caused by the use of the information given herein

Printed in Great Britain
by Amazon